EFFORT
A BEHAVIORAL NEUROSCIENCE PERSPECTIVE ON THE WILL

EFFORT
A BEHAVIORAL NEUROSCIENCE PERSPECTIVE ON THE WILL

Jay Schulkin
Department of Physiology and Biophysics
Center for Brain Basis of Cognition,
Georgetown University

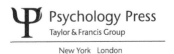
Psychology Press
Taylor & Francis Group

New York   London

First published by
Lawrence Erlbaum Associates, Inc., Publishers
10 Industrial Avenue
Mahwah, New Jersey 07430

This edition published 2012 by Psychology Press

Psychology Press   Psychology Press
Taylor & Francis Group   Taylor & Francis Group
711 Third Avenue   27 Church Road
New York, NY 10017   Hove, East Sussex BN3 2FA

Library of Congress Cataloging-in-Publication Data

Schulkin, Jay.
Effort : a behavioral neuroscience perspective on the will /
  Jay Schulkin.
      p. cm.
Includes bibliographical references and index.
ISBN 0-8058-6009-6 (cloth : alk. paper)
ISBN 0-8058-6010-X (pbk. : alk. paper)
1. Brain-Physiology. 2. Motivation. I. Title.
[DNLM: 1. Brain–physiology. 2. Motivation. WL 300 S386e
  2006]
QP376.S355 2006
612.8'2—dc22   2006011934
                                    CIP

*Dedicated to Heidi Byrnes, Micah Leshem,
and Hal Pashler*

Contents

Preface

The diverse senses of effort are fundamentally linked to motivation, behavioral inhibition, self-regulation, and "staying the course" for long-term goals despite short-term seduction. One neurotransmitter that underlies the diverse senses of effort is dopamine; this is made apparent in Parkinson's patients, but it is also apparent in most of our everyday activities, whether we are still (e.g., solving a problem in our head) or moving about.

The core thesis is twofold: Central dopamine underlies diverse tasks, and there is no absolute separation of the cognitive and noncognitive brain; there are diverse cognitive systems many of which are embodied in motor systems that underlie self-regulation.

The scientific literature abounds with studies of decision making and effort. One approach is to demythologize our understanding of cognitive systems; the effort that we exert when we think, and either move or not move through space with our bodies, reflects the cognitive machinations in the brain; aberrations of brain systems reflect the breakdown in the long- and sometimes short-term goals that serve our well-being.

The classical pragmatists have had a significant influence on my thinking and my work. William James, for example, emphasized the importance of the effort within a psychobiological context and the feeling of effort as an important part of our experience. James places the understanding of the will within the context of the organization of action.

This book cuts across disciplinary lines. As always, I thank my family, friends, and colleagues for their help.

Introduction:
Self-Preservation and Effort

The 17th-century philosopher Spinoza (1688, 1955) put it this way: "Everything ... endeavors to persist in its own being" (p. 136; see also Heidegger, 1979; Nietzsche, 1883/1961). Effort or the will is the striving that everyone experiences; it is often a state of unrest and disquiet (Schopenhauer, 1818/1958). In small children, for example, a will to live—striving and stretching, responding to discrepancies and salience—is readily apparent (Kagan, Kearsley, & Zelazo, 1978, 1980).

Darwin (1859/1958), of course, emphasized self-preservation and survival. The fight to stay alive and the origins of our intelligence are at the heart of our evolution, both biological and cultural.

Effort is a term closely associated with motivation; *will* is traditionally linked to the effector systems tied to one's goals and intentions. But in fact, effort is tied to one's goals and intentions. Although these two terms are not identical, there is sufficient overlap for my purposes that in the context of this book they will often, though not always, be used interchangeably. What do I mean by effort or the will? One recurring feature of what I have in mind is staying the course. Staying the course, staying steadfast to what one wants requires energy, power—effort or willpower. The athlete awakens to swim at 4 a.m., tired but committed to a longer term goal of competing and winning, or placing well. The structure of her life is oriented toward that end. She wants to go back to sleep, but she perseveres.

WILLIAM JAMES—DIVERSE SENSE OF EFFORT

The will, as James (1890/1952) suggests, permeates motor systems: "The will appears in every muscle as irritability" (vol. 2, p. 252). By irritability, I take it, he should mean just activation, which might entail motivation and approach behaviors, behavioral inhibition, restraint, and limiting choice and action, all of which reflect *cognitive systems* that underlie behavior.

Striving in muscular activity is phylogenetically ancient; therefore, one fundamental sense of the will is expressed in evolution through bodily expression—basic strivings. From a biological point of view, the issue has been addressed as a craving for life, a desire to persevere.

James (1897) characterizes effort and the will in terms of anticipatory cognitive regulation of motor systems (chap. 3; Elsner & Hommel, 2001; Evarts, 1973) in the context of the burgeoning conception of neuronal functions. I suggest in later chapters, and have adumbrated here, that cognition need not be separate from motor control; there is no absolute separation of the cognitive systems from the motor systems. Many motor "type" functions are tied to cognitive expression (syntax production) and a number of traditional motor areas are now known to be tied to cognitive functions (parts of the basal ganglia; Parent, 1996; Ullman, 2004).

The "kinesthetic idea," as James liked to put it, is basic to our concept of the will. The use of bodily force and the feeling of effort were critical markers of the will. The continued ability to resist or to pursue is a marking of the will—a body extended in space (Bain 1859/1886; Dooley, 2001; Ingvar, 1994). James outlined a view in which the sense of the will was knotted to diverse forms of action (Kane, 1995)—cognitive systems no less than overt behaviors (Frese & Sabini, 1985; Frijda, 1986; Gollwitzer, 1996; Jabre & Salzsieder, 1997; Spence & Frith, 1999). Effort, I suggest, is just one feature of what might be associated with the will, and even that might vary depending on the task (Fig. I.1)

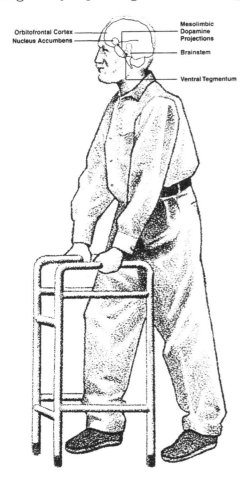

FIG. I.1. Effort in one of its many forms: battling Parkinson's Disease.

James, who was trained as a physician and taught psychology, was aware of the advances in the biological and neural sciences, and his philosophical orientation reflected these facts. James (1890/1952) made reference to the findings of Darwin and Jackson, Ferrier and Lamarck. He understood that bodily reactions—or simple reflexes, as Dewey (1896), his fellow pragmatist, also noted—are replete with ideation: ideas embodied in bodies in action. Minds are not spectators on the sidelines. This is what James and others (e.g., Lotze, 1852; see also Jeannerod, 1994) called "idea-motor" reflex. In other words, cognitive systems pervade human action, and human action is permeated by diverse goals (Prinz, 2003).

In one of his early books on psychology, John Dewey (1887/1975), like many other investigators to the present day, characterized the will as "directed towards the attainment of a recognized end which is felt as desirable" (p. 309). The will is the primary effector organ of our ideas. James (1899/1958), like many others, emphasized "the higher centers" of the brain and their importance "to exert a constant inhibitive influence" (p. 118).

EFFORT AND CONFLICT

Functional neural circuits evolved to serve diverse functions that underlie the organization of our experience and our ability to adapt to our surroundings. Our ability to sustain actions with effort, both appetitive and aversive; is a consideration of the will. The brain is the organ for this basic feature of our experiences.

Conflict is an inherent part of human action, and the will is tied to our ability to sustain actions with effort to withstand short-term, seductive gains at the expense of long-term losses, and to persevere in the face of abject adversity. Conflict tests our willpower to preserve our longer term goals.

Our evolution is inexorably bound up with the evolution of the neocortex (Jackson, 1882/1958; James, 1890/1952). Corticalization of function is a fundamental trajectory of the central nervous system that entails both syntax in language and basic motor control. Having basic motor programs under the direction of the forebrain is a feature of our evolution (Jackson, 1882/1958; James, 1890/1952), and a feature of higher order cognitive systems (Ullman, 2001). The neuroscientist Paus (2001) put it nicely: "Overcoming inertia when initiating actions and fighting competing well established or innate tendencies are two cornerstones of the willed control of behavior" (p. 422). It is corticalization of function that underlies the cognitive control over our actions.

Regions of the neocortex, particularly the frontal and anterior cingulate cortex, underlie the adjudication of conflict, of desires and behavioral options competing for expression; thus, in experiments in which, for example, blood flow is measured (positron emission tomography [PET]) in a context in which information is incongruent, there is greater blood flow within these areas (Pardo, Pardo, Janer, & Raichie, 1990). This same region of the brain is an important interface in which motor control and motivation converge with generating plans and expectations (Paus, 2001; Shidara & Richmond, 2002; Wang et al., 2005). This region of the brain is closely tied to diverse cortical regions, including frontal cortex and with reciprocal projections to and from the spinal cord (Swanson, 2000a, 2003). This region is a major target of dopamine projections from the brainstem. Both the cortical-cortical connectivity and the cortical spinal projections suggest the importance of this region in the organization of action and the expression of effort.

In other studies using single neuronal recording, the anterior cingulate cortex was particularly active during focused attention, conflict, and the generation through, in part, its connectivity with prefrontal cortex, of behavioral response selection (e.g., Isomura, Ito, Akazawa, Nambu, & Takada, 2003; Kerns et al., 2004). And in diverse studies, using PET to measure brain activity in humans, the cingulate cortex is activated, in particular, under conflict conditions (e.g., Erickson et al., 2003; Kerns et al., 2004). It is during conflict having to do with choice, with existential moments of having and coping with competing interests, that the will is most focused, balancing competing interests and staying the course; the greater the alternatives, the greater the activation of regions of the cingulate and prefrontal cortex (e.g., Kerns et al., 2004; Paus, 2001; Suchan et al., 2005; Fig. I.2). Thus, in one experiment, the greater the conflict in adjusting and monitoring a decision (and the greater the conflict) the greater the cingulate cortex is activated, as is the recruitment of cognitive control by the prefrontal cortex (e.g., Badre & Wagner, 2004; Gehring & Fenesik, 2001; Kerns et al., 2004).

One can be sure that the anterior cingulate or prefrontal cortex are not the only regions of the brain activated under conflict conditions (e.g., Greene, Sommerville, Nystrom, & Cohen, 2001; Mesulam, 1998). What we do know is that the recognition of conflict or a discrepancy is associated with attempts to adjudicate the conflict and the will has to do with managing the trajectory toward the goals that are intended (Peirce, 1878/1992a, 1877/1992d).

CONCLUSION

Perhaps our mind/brain comes prepared to use the concept of the will in understanding human choice and the evolution of accountability for our actions. Moreover, our cognitive capacity is grounded in action, and effort is a subset of our depiction of an action, as is the attribution of the will. This figures importantly in sustaining behavioral inhibition, adjudicating choices among rewards, binding oneself to future behaviors

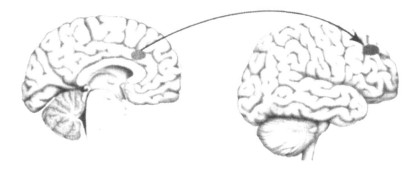

FIG. I.2.   Detection of conflict and organized control involving the cingulate and frontal cortex (Kerns et al., 2004; Matsumoto & Tanaka, 2004).

based on present expectations (Ainslie, 2001; Elster, 1979, 2000; Rachlin, 2000).

Effort is involved in:

1. Choice
2. Motivation
3. Inhibition
4. Regulation of rewards
5. Self-binding behaviors
6. Limiting the breakdown of the organization of action

The book is organized as follows: Chapter 1 is a perspective on behavioral neuroscience and the organization of effort and the will, followed in chapter 2 by a discussion of motivation and the regulation of the internal milieu. Chapter 3 promotes an understanding of the neural organization of cognitive/motor control of behavior and chapter 4 presents the sense of effort that underlies behavioral inhibition. The aberrations of our decision making via neurological afflictions are discussed in chapter 5, and the fundamental link between choice, effort, and sustained actions is explored in chapter 6.

1 Neuroscience and Interdisciplinary Inquiry

The neural sciences, though quite young, have dramatically altered the intellectual landscape during the past 50 years. From the time of the formation of the Institute of Neurological Sciences, for example, at the University of Pennsylvania in 1953, the neural sciences have been interdisciplinary. The institute was the brainchild of Louis Flexner, a biochemist who had done work in the area of memory formation. Louis Flexner, nephew of Abraham and Simon Flexner, understood that this new branch of science would require biologists, chemists, anatomists, psychologists, and psychiatrists, and the institute's faculty accordingly represented this broad spectrum of experts drawn from throughout the university (Fig. 1.1). The Institute of Neurological Sciences was to set the context for a number of other such institutes and departments of neuroscience that were to emerge in the succeeding 50 years (Morrison, 1982).

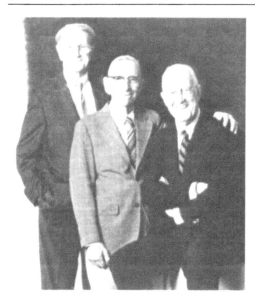

FIG. 1.1.   Three early Directors of the Institute of Neurological Sciences at the University of Pennsylvania: Louis Flexner (middle), James Sprague, and Eliot Stellar (sitting, 1991).

Eliot Stellar (in Fig. 1.1) had written the classic article on "The Physiology of Motivation" (Stellar, 1954, 1960). The concept of motivation is knotted to effort and forms the basis for the origins of what we call the will (chap. 2). The study of motivational systems, like most other behavioral studies, is inherently interdisciplinary and found a home, at that time, in the neurosciences.

Why should the study of neuroscience be so interdisciplinary? The study of the mind means, in part, studying the brain. In the 1970s, philosophical questions were focused on how to characterize the mind in the neural sciences. The idea that the mind is nothing more than neurons, in any language imaginable, is still a scientific dream, a good dream, better to discern functional relationships between mental functions and physical realizations (c. f. Block, 1978; Descombes, 2001; Hebb, 1949; Parrott & Schulkin, 1993; Weissman, 2002). Simplicity in science and elsewhere is a virtue, and a thing of beauty. But simplicity, though a normative goal, is no end.

In this chapter, I orient the reader to the general themes of the book, namely, the emphasis of mind as part of biological adaptation, cognitive systems being endemic to the organization of action, and the fundamental role of central dopamine in the organization of action and thought.

MIND AND BIOLOGY

The brain is a biological organ. We know that cognitive subsystems in the brain are diverse and recruit neural systems across the neural axis from brain stem to cortex (Gazzaniga, 2000; McCulloch & Pitts, 1943; Miller, Galanter, & Pribram, 1960). Thus, the issue is: How do subsystems in the brain perform their functions to produce what we perceive as the actions of the mind? In this regard, a certain amount of reasonable progress has been made over a short period of time. The mind is less a thing, as James (1890/1952) noted, than a collection of embodied behavioral functions. There is often no single physical entity in the brain that corresponds directly to, and is isomorphic with, a mental function. It is one thing to assert that all mental functions are embodied in neural tissue; it is another to conclude that anything that one means by a "mental function" is exhausted in the description of neuronal activity.

The brain has both broad and narrow circuits that have allowed for diverse behavioral adaptations. An example of one of the most important of these adaptations in humans is language (Chomsky, 1972; Pinker, 1994, 1998; Rozin, 1976, 1998). Most concepts, such as "motivation" or "firmness of purpose," (Lamarck, 1809/1984) or the will, do not have a direct reference to neural structure, but this does not undermine their validity. The will as an expression of the cognitive organization of action is central to understanding who we are as individuals.

To understand the brain and the mind, to understand the organization of action in people and the will, is, in part, to understand a number of specialized mechanisms that evolved to endow us with problem-solving abilities. Information processing means engagement in the everyday sense of trying to figure out what to do and how to understand an event. What is outstanding about the mind/brain is the simplicity of such complex operations.

In the past 10 years within the neurosciences and the cognitive sciences, there has been a resurgence of interest in reenvisioning the body (e.g., Damasio, 1994, 1999; Schulkin, 2004). This new view holds that cognitive systems are endemic to broad-based bodily functions and that the mind is no longer on one side and bodily functions on the other. Cognitive capacity also permeates our considerations of the motor systems. Motor control and expression and cognitive capacity are not separate or opposed to each other; they are embedded within one another. The organization of the motor system, long a neuroscientific object of study (Nauta & Freitag, 1986; Swanson, 2000b; 2003), is integrated with cognitive functions (Georgopoulos, 1994, 2000; Graybiel, Aosaki, Flaherty, & Kimura, 1994; Knowlton, Mangels, & Squire, 1996; Lieberman, 2000; Linas, 2001; Ullman, 2004).

As Lakoff and Johnson (1999) suggest, "brains tend to optimize" and "the embodiment of reason via the sensorimotor system is of great importance. It is a crucial part of the explanation of why it is possible for our concepts to fit so well with the way we function in the world" (p. 41). Cognitive systems pervade all that we do as human beings. There is no one part of the brain that is purely sensory or motor that does not have a cognitive component. There are still, nonetheless, motor and sensory and integrative neurons. One just recognizes, perhaps, that cognition is not on one side of the equation and sensory and motor events on the other.

There are diverse ways in which cognitive systems underlie our sense of action, of effort—the doing and perceiving of things. Lakoff and Johnson (1999) indicated the following:

1. Representing as doing
2. Communicating as showing
3. Searching as knowing
4. Imagining as moving
5. Attempting to gain knowledge as searching
6. Becoming aware as noticing
7. Impediments to knowledge as impediments to vision

These events are all cognitive and can require effort, resolute purpose, and staying toward a goal (e.g., searching as knowing [Heelan & Schulkin, 1998]). On the neural side, evidence suggests that performing an action and looking at another perform it can activate many of the same neural systems (e.g., Buccino et al., 2004; Decety & Grèzes, 1999; Jeannerod, 1985, 1988; Rizzolatti, Fogassi, & Gallese, 2000). The sight of others, watching them and discerning their intentions, plans, and goals activates something Jackson and Decety (2004) call "motor cognition." One recent study, interestingly, has shown that words about action (e.g., looking at action words) and the action itself activate human motor and premotor cortex. In an fMRI (functional magnetic resonance imaging) to measure brain activity, subjects were shown action words or were asked to perform a simple action. The study found that in addition to other cortical areas, motor and premotor cortex are activated by the sight of these words or the action itself (Hauk, Johnsrude, & Pulvermuller, 2004; see also Martin & Chao, 2001; Fig. 1.2). In other words, the sight of the word is enough to activate motor and premotor areas linked to the movements themselves. Cognitive systems (looking at a word) are

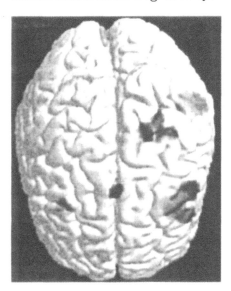

FIG. 1.2. Action words activate frontal-central motor regions (as well as other cortical sites; Hauk et al., 2004). Reprinted from *Neuron, 41,* G. Hauk, I. Johnsrude, & F. Pulvermaller, Somatotropic representation of action words in human motor and premotor cortex, 301–307, copyright © 2004, with permission from Elsevier.

inherent in cortical (and perhaps subcortical, basal ganglia) motor systems.

CHEMICAL CODING, NEURAL CIRCUITS, AND BEHAVIOR

Dopamine is a fundamental neurotransmitter that underlies the organization of effort and the will, and that figures in virtually every chapter of this book. Dopamine is a catecholamine and is produced in the adrenal gland and in core structures of the brain (Fig. 1.3). It is an ancient molecule that underlies di-

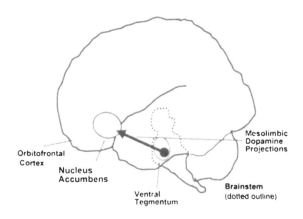

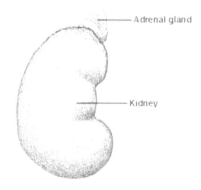

FIG. 1.3. Dopamine in the brain, and dopamine from the adrenal gland.

verse behavioral functions. Dopamine is just one neurotransmitter among others (this will be repeated), but it is an important one for the organization of cognitive systems and for action (Cools & Robbins, 2004; Dreisbach et al., 2005).

Dopamine is a fundamental neurotransmitter for diverse cognitive functions, for example, language (Ullman, 2001); and probability computations (Schultz, 2002); it is fundamental also in the organization of drive and reward (Hoebel, 1998). It may be fundamental in the development of behavioral inhibition (Diamond, 2001). Both excess and depletion of this transmitter are reflected in diverse forms of pathology (e.g., Parkinson's disease). The regulation of this transmitter, for behavior, is a fundamental event.

Dopamine, as well as serotonin and norepinephrine, are amines. They are represented in specific neuronal sites in the brain stem and forebrain (e.g., Brown et al., 1976, 1979). From small clusters of cell bodies, a diverse array of fiber pathways connects to a large part of the brain; this is true of all the amines (e.g., dopamine; Mogenson, Yang, Yim, 1991; Simon, Scatton, & LeMoal, 1980; Spanagel and Weiss, 1999). For example, dopaminergic pathways from the substantia nigra innervate the putamen and caudate nucleus of the striatum (Swanson, 1988, 2000a, 2000b). This is the nigrostriatal system, which is involved in subcortical motor control. Dysfunction of this system is associated with certain movement disorders, such as Parkinson's disease (Parkinson, 1817) and tardive dyskinesia (Marsden, Merton, Adam, & Hallet, 1978). The initiation of movement and the organization of thought are important functions of the nigrostriatal system and are illustrated by the characteristics of Parkinson's disease (Marsden, Merton, Adam, & Hallet, 1978; Marsden & Obeso, 1994). In other words, there are diverse kinds of data that associate a decrease of cognitive performance along with the well- known movement impairments in Parkinson's disease (e.g., Mochi et al., 2004).

The mesocorticolimbic dopamine system includes the brain systems that are important for the ingestion of food, water, drugs, and social and other rewards (Berridge & Robinson, 1998; Kelley, 1999, 2004; Spanagel & Weiss,

1999; Wise, 2005; Worsley et al., 2000). This system can be subdivided into two systems, the mesolimbic system and the mesocortical system. The mesolimbic system consists of dopaminergic projections from the midbrain ventral tegmental area to the limbic forebrain areas, including the nucleus accumbens, stria terminalis, lateral septal nuclei, amygdala, and limbic areas of the striatum (Brodal, 1981; Spanagel & Weiss, 1999, 2005; Swanson, 2000a, 2000b). In the mesocortical dopamine system, the dopamine cell bodies are also located in the ventral tegmental area. Subsets of dopaminergic projections terminate in the prefrontal cortex, anterior cingulate, and entorhinal cortex (Tzchentke, 2000).

Dopamine levels are linked to diverse motivated behaviors (e.g., Kelley, 1999, 2004). These links have led a number of investigators to connect dopamine to reward (e.g., Becker et al., 2001; Hollerman et al., 2000; Lucas, Pompei, & McEwen, 2000; Spanagel & Weiss 1999; Tzchentke, 2001). But dopamine neurons are activated under a number of diverse conditions, including duress. Dopamine, like the other amines in the brain, is also essential for the broad-based coordination for adaptive responses and is tied to the organization of thought and action, central to both the activation of behavior and the inhibition of behavior. Dopamine is neutral with regard to function; it is just essential for the organization of behavior, the organization of effort (e.g., solving a math problem, running, persevering, inhibiting behavior).

Dopamine is a broadly based neurotransmitter with a number of receptors that are regulated by different transcription factors. Dopamine is one neurotransmitter that is closely linked to the concept of the will. It underlies the feeling of effort, the organization of action, and the rational prioritizing of our goals. The important thing to note at the onset is the hypothesis that dopamine is neutral; dopamine is active, I suggest, under both positive and negative conditions. It is essential to have dopamine elevated and regulated during the organization of thought and the organization of action, not just during positive reward or the inhibition of behavior.

CONCLUSION

Our sense of effort figures in the consideration of motivation, behavioral inhibition, delayed gratification, and decision making. These core features are knotted to, what James and Dewey called *the feeling of effort*. The sense of effort is tied to motivational systems, to central states of the brain. This may require understanding cognitive systems as not separate from motor systems.

Athletic experiences are one example of the exercise of effort—a serious competitive swimmer is a paradigmatic example of perseverance despite adversity, staying the course, and most definitely experiencing the sense of effort. Of course, the athlete has to balance a sense of reward with the pain that they might be experiencing (Fig. 1.4). They have to withstand short-term discomfort, and set their sights on anticipatory and longer term satisfaction (Ainslie, 2001; Sterling, 2004). The contents of each of the chapters that follow will figure in

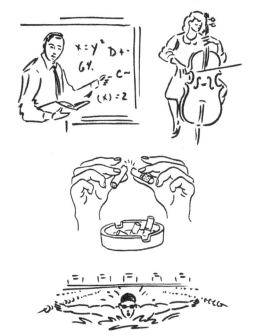

FIG. 1.4. Diverse contexts in which the will is manifest.

explaining the athlete's behavior; the effort and motivation, the cognitive control embedded in neural design, the focus and attention that is required, the inhibition of competing interests, the visualization of action, and the good fortune of possessing a certain temperament.

2 Central Motive States

Motivated systems are orchestrated by cognitive and neural devices, some of which are flexible in design structure (Gallistel, 1980,1992). Forebrain regions modulate the expression of behavioral outputs and adjudicate conflicting appetites and desires. Central behavioral programs figure in the expression of motivated behaviors (Swanson, 2000a; 2005).

This chapter will begin by conveying a basic feature of animal life, namely, perseverance and survival. Motivational systems and their evolution figures in our understanding of the origins of effort and the will and with the regulation of the internal milieu and stability. We know that diverse cognitive systems underlie sensory motor control in motivational systems and that dopamine is vital in the organization of motivation, action, and problem solving.

EVOLUTION: SURVIVAL AND STRIVING TO PERSEVERE

Evolutionary theory did not begin with Charles Darwin, but it was never the same afterward. Evolutionary concepts were in the intellectual air that Darwin breathed. They leaked from the pens of Lyell, Erasmus, Darwin, and Malthus (see Gould, 2002).

Competition, speciation, strife, and resolution were beginning to be understood as part of the regulatory events of nature. The will was always linked to power, which was a vital fact of the animal kingdom of living things and of vital forces; a fundamental intuition about us is the sense of willing something into existence (e.g., Bergson, 1913/2001; James, 1890/1952).

Lamarck (1809/1984) was well-known for the idea that the mechanism by which natural selection operated could be illustrated in the example of giraffes. Lamarck thought that giraffes' long necks evolved because the animals stretched them to reach food in high tree canopies and then passed on this physical trait to the next generation. Less well known is the fact that Darwin (1871, 1874) also believed that serviceable habits were inherited.

An early evolutionary perspective on the origins and development of self-regulation was tied to "spontaneous generation" in the language of Lamarck (1809/1984). Lamarck understood that the brain was the vital organ for the formation of willful acts. He understood that "the nervous system of the most perfect animals ... [has] special faculties" (p. 298) and noted those "wrinkled hemispheres" (p. 309) and their enlargement. This enlargement of the cortex is fundamental for self-regulation. The will is placed in a functional context. Lamarck also noted "that animals which have no nervous system cannot possess the faculty of will" (p. 357). Nature was forced to "add a new organ to the nervous system" (p. 358). The important point is that the power to express one's interest reveals the will.

The heart of evolution, as Darwin (1859/1958) stated in his great work *On the Origin of Species*, is "never to forget that every single organic being may be said to be striving the utmost to increase in numbers; that each lives by a struggle at some period of its life" (p. 77). Perhaps Spinoza (1688/1958), a more modern stoic philosopher, was prescient several centuries earlier—from the pantheon of pantheism and rationalism—when he asserted that all living things struggle to persevere.

Darwin spent a lot of textual time referring to the development of habits for behavioral adaptation. He noted that "when our minds are much affected, so are the movements of our bodies" (1872/1998, p. 32). The will, put in more modern terms, can be understood as a piece of cognitive/behavioral adaptation. What function does it serve? Surely it brings about the ends that we are trying to achieve, therefore permeating many of our adaptations, needs, strivings, and both proximate and long-term ends. Effort is required in our ability to regulate our behaviors elicited by motivations and conflicted needs for the consideration of long-term goals. In other words, we act, or, rather, can exercise our behavioral strivings, in relation to a cognitive arsenal that includes principles under which our persistence is, in principle, legitimated.

Darwin (1871, 1874) refers to the will in terms of control. He says, "The highest possible stage in moral culture is when we recognize that we ought to control our thoughts" (p. 119). The descent into barbarism, for this Victorian, as for many of us, is the absence of regulation of our thoughts and actions. Behavioral regulation is vital as an expression of the will. The will is particularly relevant in the origins of self-determination. This is probably what Darwin had in mind, in part, by the preceding statement.

BEHAVIORAL REGULATION OF THE INTERNAL MILIEU

Animals strive to persevere; they are motivated. To be motivated is to be willing to generate effort to achieve a goal. Motivation is, by definition, linked to goals and expectations (Hinde, 1970; Teitelbaum, 1971; Tolman, 1932).

Representations of actions underlie motivation and drives (Stellar, 1954; Stellar & Corbit, 1973). Motivation reflects a wide variety of factors: physiological needs, hedonic assessment, learning, and history. Although instincts have long been linked to drives and motivational systems (Lorenz, 1965, 1981), they are not identical to such systems. The concepts of drive and motivation are larger than the innate, specific, fixed action patterns that were selected by natural selection (Epstein, 1982; Flynn, 1972; Thorndike, 1935; Thorpe, 1963; Tinbergen, 1951).

In fact, central motive states are a fundamental property of the nervous system (Lashley, 1938; Stellar, 1954), and a number of specific and generic motivational systems pervade the nervous system (e.g., thirst, hunger, sex, safety, and closeness). Central motive states are states that underlie approach and avoidance behavioral responses, the integration of coherent behavioral expression, the activation of perceptual/learning, and systems that underlie the information processing systems in the brain. Simple drive reductions are not sufficient to explain motivational systems, for diverse animals are driven by diverse incentives, but drives are an important component of the scope of the concept of motivation (Berridge, 2004; Toates, 1986; Fig. 2.1).

Motivation functions across a wide domain of information-processing systems (Gallistel, 1980). But the concept of motivation, like that of will, is tied to our considerations of generating sufficient energy to achieve those goals.

The maintenance of the internal milieu is one key factor on the biological side of motivational systems (Fig. 2.2). Animals strive through behavioral means to maintain internal viability. Behavior, like physiology, serves to maintain short- and long-term adaptation, and motivational systems serve this end. Physiological actions are based on, and cannot exist independently of, cognitive structure and processing—in fact, it can be argued that cognitive physiology is the foundation of

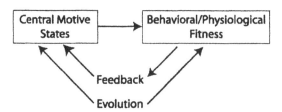

FIG. 2.1. Expression of central motive states.

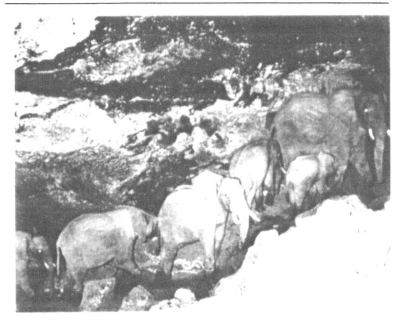

FIG. 2.2.   Elephants are known to search and remember where salt licks are to be found. Here is one elephant at a salt lick (photo courtesy of Ian Redmond).

motivational systems (Gallistel, 1980). Remembering where water and salt are to be found when one is hungry for water and salt (Krieckhaus & Wolf, 1968) is but one example in which motivational systems are bound to and not separate from cognitive structures and functions in the brain.

For example, a whole new level of complexity was added, not only to physiology but also to evolutionary ascent, by the ability to maintain the balance of body fluid amid changes in external and internal conditions through the central regulation of behavior (Richter, 1927, 1947). The great degree to which physiological systems are devoted to the maintenance of the internal milieu and physiological viability (e.g., Cannon, 1929) has been established. Behavioral motivations evolved to serve both short- and long-term goals (e.g., reproductive success)—thus did motivational systems spiral into a variety of behavioral shapes.

Studies in laboratory rats show that a chronic loss of bodily sodium leads to increased ingestion of the mineral (Richter,

1927, 1947). In nature, sodium-hungry animals seek out sodium, and domesticated animals (e.g., horses) ingest sodium as needed when it is freely offered (Denton, 1982). Sodium-starved laboratory rats will press a bar (Wolf, 1969) and will run down runways to receive sodium (Schulkin, Arnell, & Stellar, 1985; Fig. 2.3). A hedonic shift is partly responsible for ensuring that sodium will be ingested, even if normally aversive concentrations of sodium (e.g., seawater) are all that is available. Sodium-hungry rats, which reject and display unpleasant facial expressions in response to hypertonic sodium infusions into the oral cavity, when not sodium sated, will accept the solution and even show facial expressions like those seen when ingesting sucrose (Berridge, Flynn, Schulkin, & Grill, 1984). The motivation to seek out and ingest salt solutions in sodium-hungry animals is thus partly based on a change in what is deemed to be palatable with regard to salt solutions.

Ingestion is a behavior that is influenced both by external motivational pulls, in the form of, for example, what other tastes sodium is associated with and where it can be found, and by the internal bodily drives of the animal (Krieckhaus, 1970; Schulkin 1991; Wolf, 1969). Interestingly, the hormones that raise the motivation to search and ingest sodium

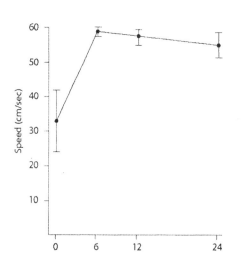

FIG. 2.3. Speed of running for hypertonic NaCl at various concentrations (0% = water) in a runway by sodium-hungry rats; note that sodium-hungry rats will run for NaCl at concentrations above what they are willing to consume (e.g., 24%). Reprinted from *Hormones and Behavior*, *19*, J. Schulkin, P. Arnell, & E. Stellar, Running to the taste of salt in mineralocorticoids treated rats, 413–425, copyright © 1985, with permission from Elsevier.

(e.g., Denton, 1982; Fitzsimons, 1999; Fluharty, 2002) also increase central dopamine levels (Frankmann et al., 1994; Lucas et al., 2000, 2003). From a biological point of view, behavior serves the internal milieu to achieve bodily viability both in the short term and the long term (i.e., reproductive success). Diverse central motivate states are linked to the regulation of internal milieu are tied to reward (e.g., Berridge, 2004; Stellar, 1954, 1960). One area of the brain that has now been linked to reward is the basal ganglia; neurons in the ventral pallidal region are activated to the enhanced hedonic value of NaCl (sodium chloride) when the rats are sodium hungry (Smith et al., 2004).

The treatment of motivational systems and the selection of one behavioral pattern over another has often been couched in terms of "spontaneity of behavior" (Epstein, 1982; Teitelbaum, 1971). I think this is an unfortunate use of words (e.g., Bergson, 1913/2001). According to this view, motivational systems are always flexible and voluntary. This is misleading and incorrect. The motivational system can be both mechanical and diverse in expression. The sharp contrast between the mechanical and the spontaneous and creative is undercut by our reasoning about biological systems. We need to reenvision our notion of the mechanical. But surely mechanisms are not one-sided, that is, either dead and inert or dynamic, lifelike, and free. Biological systems, motivational systems in which considerations of the will are to be found in behavioral striving for short- and long-term satisfaction, undercut this distinction between dynamism and the mechanical; the contrast was between that which was considered dynamic and free or extended spatially and that which was determined (e.g., Bergson, 1913/2001).

Not all agree that concepts such as motivation are legitimate in our scientific lexicon. The principle of parsimony can eliminate the concept (Dethier, 1982). The concept of motivation can be eliminated from the vernacular of scientific respectability and use, or it can be easily abused and used in a viciously circular manner (see Wise, 1987, for a critique of the concept of motivation). More sanguine positions render the concept an intervening variable (Miller, 1948, 1959). I am a *realist* about the concept of motivation; what do I mean? Motivation is vital in the explanation of behavior and is a fundamental property of very diverse animals (e.g., Berridge, 2004; Morgan & Stellar, 1950; Peters, 1958, 1975; Stellar & Stellar, 1985; Toates, 1986).

In other words, the concept of motivation is a key category in our mental lexicon. Motivation is fundamental in the organization of action embodied in neural structure. It is a key category in the prediction and explanation of actions, a real property of our brain. Moreover, fundamental features of motivation include appetitive and consummatory behaviors (Craig, 1918; Dewey, 1925/1989). The approach and the consummatory expression of motivation behaviors (e.g., the labor to find sodium and the satisfaction with its consumption; Berridge et al., 1984) is an example of rooted biological behaviors.

SENSORY/MOTOR INTEGRATION, DOPAMINE, AND MOTIVATIONAL SYSTEMS

Sensory motor integration is essential for motivation. Both specific and general neural circuits underlie motivational systems. Specific drives (e.g., sex, water, food, sodium, etc.) have specific interceptive signals that interact with competing interests and external contexts for expression. Motivational expression does not take place in a vacuum; it occurs in environments in which animals are adapting, or not.

The nucleus accumbens, which is part of the basal ganglia, is a major area in the organization of action (Nauta & Domesick, 1982; Nauta, Smith, Faull, & Domesick, 1978). The nucleus accumbens is part of the circuitry by which motivational interceptive signals (desired goals that underlie behavior) from hypothalamus and amygdala is transduced into motor output and behavior (Graybiel, 2001; Kelley, 2004; Mogenson, Jones, & Yim, 1980; Swanson & Mogenson, 1981). More generally regions of the striatum and are now well known to underlie appetitive motivation—dopamine expression plays an important role in the organization appetitive of behaviors (Ikemoto & Panksepp, 1999; Kelley, 2004).

Dopamine plays an important role in diverse forms of generating motivated behaviors.

The neurotransmitter dopamine is fundamental in the organization of movement and in the control of sensory information (Marshall, Richardson, & Teitelbaum, 1974; Marshall, Turner, & Teitelbaum, 1971) that is essential for the organization of action. Depletion of this fundamental neurotransmitter compromises behavioral competence and sensory/motor integration (Ungerstedt, 1971), which contain the basic ingredients for behavioral control. Lesions of the lateral hypothalamus, which decrease central dopamine, impair sensory motor and motivational functions (Marshall et al., 1971; 1974). In the laboratory, decreases in dopamine levels are associated with lethargy in performing operant responses, while elevated levels are associated with increases in effort. Decreased levels of dopamine reduce a wide variety of motivated behaviors that are linked to the regulation of the internal milieu (food, water and salt intake, sexual behavior, etc.; Stricker & Zigmond, 1974). Dopamine is essential (Marsden & Obeso, 1994) and is vital for motivational systems and for the expression of effort and the will in humans.

Consider again the example for sodium hunger. Using 6-hydroxydopamine to deplete the vast majority of central dopamine (by central injections), one observation in rats was that sodium-hungry subjects ingested far less sodium; it was concluded that the ability to integrate behavioral options and thereby ingest sodium was severely compromised by the depletion of central dopamine. But that is not to say that they would not ingest sodium (Roitman, Schafe, Thiele, & Bernstein, 1997; Stricker & Zigmond, 1974). It is just that critical central dopamine is vital for an integrated behavioral response. Interestingly, sodium depletion is known to induce structural changes in the nucleus accumbens, and the induction of such changes in the basal ganglia have been linked to other appetitive behaviors (Robinson & Kolb, 1999; Roitman, Anderson, Jones, & Bernstein, 2002; Roitman, Wheeler, & Carelli, 2005; Fig. 2.4).

The expression of central dopamine influences the attentional response to environmental information; it de-

A.

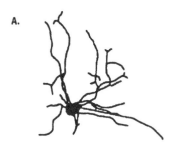

B.

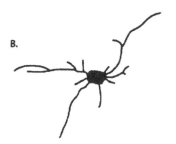

FIG. 2.4.   Representative drawings of neurons from the shell of
the nucleus accumbens, (a) from
a rat with a history of sodium depletion, and (b) from a rat with
no history of sodium depletion.
(after Roitman et al., 2002).
Copyright © 2002, reprinted by
permission of the Society for Neuroscience.

creases or increases attention to and the learning of environmental events; in other words, increased salience of
environmental information is one consequence of elevated
dopamine levels (Kelley, 2004; Schultz, 2002).

Reactive and Anticipatory Motivated Responses

One of the most adaptive features that evolved in diverse animals was behavioral and physiological anticipation of future
events. The anticipatory representation of events for James
(1890/1952) was the "forerunner of our voluntary acts" (p.
501). After all, our ability to anticipate and approach or avoid
events, that is, to strategically position ourselves, is at the
heart of our cognitive evolution. Anticipatory actions are an
evolutionary advantage and reflects different patterns of regulation by the brain.

Reactive responses are first-order adaptations in the physiological and behavioral repertoires. For example, deviation in
the biological thermostat results in behavioral and physiolog-

ical responses to return the body temperature to normal. Reactive homeostasis responds to external conditions and restores stability. Anticipation thus serves to avoid reactions that create wear and tear and that are not adaptive in the long run. In this way, harmful contexts that require extended use of energy are avoided. Similarly, cognitive mechanisms facilitate avoidance in behavioral control.

Our species (and surely others as well) became more successful as we were able to predict and anticipate events and to respond alternatively to events. Primary motivational systems are organized to either approach or avoid objects in the outside world. From simple reactions to anticipatory responses, our ability to adapt, predict, and avoid took full measure in our evolutionary ascent. The ability to control and inhibit our behavior, and then apply this control to anticipated events, is essentially related to our conception of the will.

Several regulatory concepts have emerged positing that we are reactive and anticipatory from both a behavioral and a physiological point of view. The term *predictive homeostasis* has been coined to refer to mechanisms that underlie anticipatory needs (Moore-Ede, 1986). Animals store food for future use, burn some metabolic fuels to "conserve," and change their needs in anticipation of future needs, and in each of these cases dopaminergic neurons should be activated.

Evolution favored organisms that were anticipatory, planning ahead, or that at least possessed a wide variety of mechanisms that allowed them to alter present conditions in light of future needs (Schulkin, 2003; Sterling & Eyer, 1988; Wingfield, 2004). Accelerating one physiological system, responding or not responding to signals in the interest of longer term goals, such capacities to self-regulate accelerated the evolutionary ascent of our biological systems.

Cephalic innervation of peripheral organs, and greater accessibility of cognitive functions within the brain itself (from more evolved regions to the brain stem), allowed for greater extension and use of behavior in more diverse domains of basic functions (Rozin, 1998). Anticipatory responses accrued with our evolutionary ascent. Our cognitive expansion was tied to this capacity to plan ahead, to avoid things that are harmful (rather than just escape them), and to exercise some control by avoidance of events. Not surprisingly, the prefrontal cortex and its link to diverse regions of the brain underlie our focus, our memory and purpose in the organization of action (Sterling, 2004; Fig. 2.5).

A. Neocortical cascades to prefrontal cortex   B. Limbic cascades to prefrontal cortex

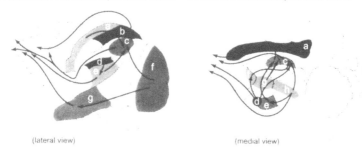

(lateral view)   (medial view)

C. Prefrontal cascades to neocortex   D. Prefrontal cascades to limbic system

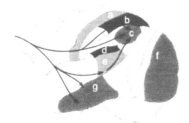
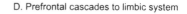
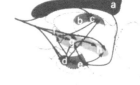

a. primary somatosensory   a. cingulate gyrus
b. secondary somatosensory   b. anterior thalamic nucleus
c. inferior parietal lobule (multimodal)   c. dorsomedial thalamic nucleus
d. primary auditory   d. amygdala
e. secondary auditory   e. hippocampus
f. primary visual   f. septum
g. secondary visual   g. hypothalamus
                                                 h. midbrain limbic area

FIG. 2.5.   Projections between the prefrontal cortex and diverse regions of the brain (Sterling, 2004).

The Concept of Motivation

The concept of motivation seems innocuous enough—try explaining behavior without it. Several years ago, my colleague Israel Lederhandler of the National Institute of Mental Health and I put together a conference titled "The Place of the Concept of Motivation in Contemporary Neuroscience." Most of the participants were silent, antagonistic, or rejecting of the legitimacy of this concept in neuroscience. Most were practicing neuroscientists, and perhaps only 3 or 4 out of 20 were committed to the concept of motivation as a legitimate category in our scientific lexicon. Most thought that motivation was a concept best left behind or at least not talked about. Why? Tracing a reflex like conditioned fear is tractable from a neuroscience perspective; motivation and related terms are much less so. They would think even less of the concept of the will.

At the conference, I asserted what is obvious for those of us in the field: We have moved beyond the concept of *motivation* as a simple hypothalamic function. The older view was that motivation was a function of lateral and ventral medial hypothalamic excitatory and inhibitory expression for motivated behaviors. At one time, a great flurry of scientific activity was centered on this hypothesis. Although motivation was not necessarily understood, much was discovered about neural function and its link to behavioral and regulatory physiology. A hypothesis can be wrong in total but can nonetheless generate many interesting and informative discoveries. We learned a lot about hypothalamic function because of the hypothesis that Eliot Stellar presented in 1954. But motivation, like the concept of the will and a wide variety of traditional mental terms, is not identical with sets of neural structures. Appetitive states, which encompass one feature of the will and are tied to motivation, are much more than hypothalamic activation, as was indicated in the original theory of Stellar. Some 30 years ago, fewer than 10 pathways to and from the hypothalamus had been identified, whereas now 10 times that number is known (Bota, Dong, & Swanson, 2003; Swanson, 2000a).

Motivation, as I have suggested, is not a concept identical with one set of brain regions. As I have indicated, the assertion that there is "no one-to-one map" means just that; a number of mental concepts can be justified by specifying the functional context in which one uses the terms; for example, the role of the hypothalamus in motivation/cognition/emotion, for the organization of action, and facilitating approach-avoidance behavioral responses is partially known (i.e., stimulation of the lateral and ventral hypothalamic sites; Stellar & Stellar, 1985). However, approach and avoidance behavioral systems, let alone the concept of motivation, do not map easily onto neural circuits that traverse cortical and brain stem areas (Davidson et al., 1990; Stellar & Stellar, 1985).

Our sense of the will emerges out of our consideration of motivated systems. We are a complex, motivated animal, with diverse and competing sets of choices to be made and decisions that need to be secured. It is within the contexts of motivation, behavioral inhibition, and choices that the concept of the will figures in our lexicon.

In other words, the rudiments for having a will lie in motivated behaviors: the ability to approach and avoid objects, to postpone rewards, and to remember and anticipate events. In fact, the mechanisms for anticipatory control over behavior, evolving in the context of motivational systems, play a fundamental role in the organization of action and the expression of the will in humans.

CONCLUSION

A central thesis of this book is that cognitive systems are endemic to the organization of behavioral systems (e.g. Gallistel, 1992). The brain, at each level of the neural axis, can be seen as a broad array of computational devices. One way—though slightly misleading—to envision the organization of motivated behaviors is in terms of reflexes: cortically mediated systems that underlie voluntary control and systems that mediate behavioral states (Swanson, 2000a, 2000b, 2003). Cognition is often identified with cortical voluntary control, and this, I submit, is misleading. Cognition can be reflexive (linguistic), and surely the mechanisms are unconscious. Cognition is endemic to the brain and to self-motivated behavior.

The ability to anticipate what resources might be available requires the cognitive capacity to plan ahead; self-regulation is one of the key features of our evolutionary ascent. Regulation of the internal milieu to maintain viability amid changing circumstances is part of the cephalic leap into peripheral and cortical–brain stem regulation. We learned to regulate ourselves and separate from the environment, to create a new environment, to push our brains and our bodies, and to embody motivational systems in diverse expressions beyond the narrowly biobehavioral.

Self-discipline is fundamental to the organization of thought and action. We often marvel at the fantastic discipline of the dancer, swimmer, and musician. Our cultural legacy demands a disciplined will under our control. Its rudiments are found in the basic biobehavioral regulatory systems that set us apart from merely reacting to environmental changes. These regulatory systems help us to anticipate, change, and avoid events. The organization of these events reflects the cognitive machinery of the brain, which is mediated by neurotransmitters such as dopamine. These neurotransmitters are essential for the sensory/motor integration that is vital in the motivation to avoid or approach objects, to stay or leave.

The chemical signature in the brain for motivated behaviors, such as the search for water and sodium, the drive for sex, and the avoidance of objects in the environment, has become better known over the past 30 years (Berridge, 2004; Herbert, 1993; Herbert & Schulkin, 2002; Hoebel, 1988). The chemical signatures are not identical to the concept of motivation, let alone the concept of the will.

Central motivation states are, in part, tied to the psychology of effort, to sensory motor integration. The evolution of our cognitive arsenal was accompanied by a greater capacity for choice and for integrating diverse needs or drives.

3 Willing to Believe: Reenvisioning Cognitive/Motor Control

James (1890/1952) was right to highlight the kinesthetic feature of our actions—the feeling of effort. Cognitive systems are pervasive in our understanding of the organization of action (e.g., Gallistel, 1980). Importantly, James and others (e.g., Dewey, 1896; Lashley, 1951; see also Prinz, 2003) understood cognitive systems as endemic to motor control. Cognitive systems underlie, and can be anticipatory of, movement. Reenvisioning the motor systems is to suggest that there is no absolute separation of the motor systems from the cognitive systems in the brain (see also Gallistel, 1992; Jackson & Decety, 2004; Kimura, 1993).

All features of the neural tissue, in some critical way (sensory, motor; Adey, 1974; Arbib, 1981; Wise, 1997), are cognitive in the sense that they involve information processing. Not separating cognitive systems from motor systems gives us a better lexicon for linking acts of will to the organization of action. If cognitive systems have to do with information processing and the organization of action, we need to move away from the view of cognition as mainly a cortical affair, and toward the view that cognition is at every level of the neural axis.

Let's begin this chapter first, with a traditional 19th-century view of sensory-motor function and the cortex, to a modern view about cognitive systems and the brain, then to the basal ganglia (head ganglia of motor control) and the idea that this motor area is involved in complex cognitive tasks, to regions of both the cortex and the basal ganglia that underlie the organization of cognitive tasks (syntax, memory, perception of others). Reenvisioning cognitive systems amid motor control is a step toward understanding something about how willing is realized in behavioral/neural systems.

SENSORY-MOTOR FUNCTIONS AND THE CORTEX

The great 19th-century neurologists uncovered some of the diverse roles of the motor cortex (e.g., Defelipe & Jones, 1988; Ferrier, 1886; Flourens, 1824; Hitzig, 1900; Von Bonin, 1960) including its role in syntax (Broca, 1863). Many of these early neurologists were oriented to what became known as "cortical excitability" (Finger, 1994, 2000). It was during this time that fundamental insights into the synapses, cortical columns, and developmental changes in cortical tissue were beginning to take shape (Cajal, 1906; Sherrington, 1893, 1906/1947; see Finger, 1994; Swanson, 2003).

Hughlings Jackson (1882/1958) in particular was quick to incorporate the insights that were beginning to emerge from evolutionary theory (see Critchley & Critchley, 1998). With his interest in understanding epileptic seizures (what was voluntary and what was not), Jackson (1863) understood that brain damage to the cortex, in effect, created de-evolution, the converse of evolution; the loss of behavioral control and options.

Representations of bodily limbs were spread out across the motor cortex. As Jackson (1882/1958) stated, "The nervous system is representing systems" (p. 41). He understood the mind/brain in simple sensory-motor terms. There were no "ghosts" in the brain, or anything other than sensory-motor function. However, cognitive systems were foreign to him and most of his contemporaries. But they had incorporated function and evolution into their concepts of the mind. A modern view of the cortical motor system is depicted in Fig. 3.1 (Rizzolatti & Luppino, 2001).

In this context, Hughlings Jackson (1882/1958; see also Finger, 1994, 2000) for example, depicted the motor cortex as being linked to voluntary motor control and the lower regions of the brain (i.e., striatum) as organizing involuntary control.

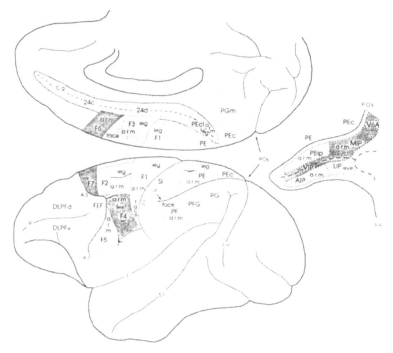

FIG. 3.1.   Medial and lateral views of the monkey brain showing the parcellation of the motor cortex, posterior parietal, and cingulate cortices. The areas located within the intraparietal sulcus are shown in an unfolded view of the sulcus in the right part of the figure. Al = inferior arcuate sulcus; AS = superior arcuate sulcus; C = central-sulcus; Cg = cingulated sulcus; DLPFd = dorsolateral prefrontal cortex, dorsal; DLPFv = dorsolateral prefrontal cortex, ventral; L = lateral fissure; Lu = lunate sulcus; P = principal sulcus; POs = parieto-occipital sulcus; ST = superior temporal sulcus. From *Neuron, 31*, G. Rizzolatti & G. Luppino, The cortical motor system, 889–901, copyright © 2001, with permission from Elsevier.

However, like many investigators of the brain, Jackson understood behavior as a chain of reflexes. The brain, we now know, generates behavior by endogenous mechanisms that are not simply a chain of sensory-motor reflexes (e.g., Lashley, 1951; Linas, 2001; Twitchell, 1954).

A number of behavioral functions are fixed and demonstrate little flexibility, whereas others are more labile (Marler & Hamilton, 1966; Preuss et al., 1996; Sumbre et al., 2001). Whether they are fixed or labile, the cognitive motor system, which is vital for the realization of the will is rich in anticipatory control. Everyday life is rife with the development of new motor habits. The development of motor control is one of the fundamental events in the nervous system, and the development of muscles, nerves, and bodies reflects endogenous processes. Endogenous processes do not take place in a vacuum, but in environments (e.g., development of song or linguistic expression; Lieberman, 2000; Marler & Hamilton, 1966), and a key component of the learning of motor tasks are the central pattern generators (Bizzi & Mussa-Ivaldi, 2000; Evarts, 1981; Humphrey & Freund, 1991; Mogenson et al., 1980; Swanson, 2003).

Basal ganglia: The basal ganglia, along with the motor cortex and to some extent the cerebellum, are fundamental in the regulation of motor control, not necessarily movement per se but the serial order of behavior. The basal ganglia are localized under the cerebral cortex and are composed of the striatum, which consists of the caudate and the putamen, in addition to another region called the globus pallidus (Alexander et al., 1991; Alheid & Heimer, 1988; Kelley, 2004; Nauta & Freitag, 1986; Saper, 1996; Fig. 3.2). These regions are reciprocally connected to the frontal cortex and other cortical regions, in addition to other sites that underlie the organization of action (Saper, 1996; Swanson, 2000a). For example, the full range of cortical inputs, both new and old cortex, project into the striatum and the limbic regions, projecting in particular into the ventral striatum (Saper, 1996).

The anatomical connections between the frontal cortex and basal ganglia constitute the head cephalic representation that underlies the organization of action. Central generators are a

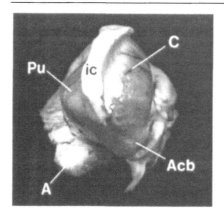

FIG. 3.2.   A view of the putamin (PU), caudate (C), and amygdala (A). ic = internal capsule (courtesy of Heimer & Alheid, unpublished).

vital source in the brain's generation of action (Swanson, 2000a, 2003; Fig. 3.3 & 3.4).

A great deal is now known about the extensive projections from this region of the brain. Nauta was a very influential neuroscientist and was important in highlighting the anatomical link between limbic contributions for motivation and organized action by stressing the role of this region of the brain (Nauta & Domesick, 1982; Nauta & Freitag, 1986). Many other investigators would expand on this insight (Graybiel, 2001; Kelley, 2004; Mogenson et al., 1980).

SENSORY-MOTOR CONTROL AND BEHAVIORAL COHERENCE

Early in human development, an infant experiences a broad array of sensory experiences, both pleasures and discomforts. She is roused by these sensory pulls to explore the world. Signals with evolutionary value were selected and help organize behavioral development (Tinbergen, 1951). The child's world, though narrow in scope, is filled with information-processing systems that are essential for taking possession of the world, for organizing oneself in relation to the objects that one might encounter (Piaget, 1952). While an earlier view emphasized the sensory side of development, newer studies point to the pervasive cognitive capabilities that underlie human development (Carey, 2004).

It is apparent that a good deal of the nervous system is devoted to sensorimotor integration, but these sensorimotor systems are integrated with cognitive information systems. The mechanisms that underlie the organization of sensorimotor functions also underlie the organization of action.

Instead of envisioning the motor system as separate from cognitive systems as traditionally understood (e.g., Mogenson et al., 1980; Swanson, 2000a, 2003), I suggest that cognitive systems are embodied in the organization of motor systems (e.g., syntax; see next section). That certainly does not mean that cognitive systems are confined to motor systems; surely they are not. In other words, there is no separation of cogni-

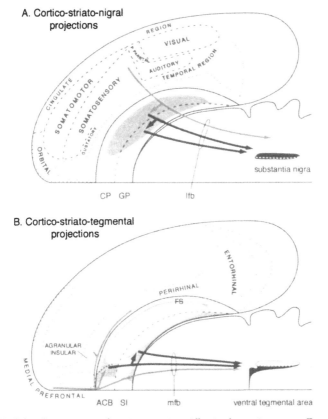

FIG. 3.3. Cortico-striatal projections to midbrain dopamine areas. From *Brain Research, 886*, L. W. Swanson, cerebral hemisphere regulation of motivated behavior, 113–164, copyright © 2000, with permission from Elsevier.

tion from motor systems; there are diverse forms of cognitive systems, some of which are tightly linked to motor control and the organization of action. I would suggest we consider that cognition is not on one side and the organization of action, its initiation, basic programming, and execution (Mogenson et al., 1980) on the other side. No one piece of the organization of action is noncognitive.

The deliberate system is associated with cognitive systems that seem more flexible, (Camerer et al., 2005). We know now that many systems are not flexible, certainly not conscious and certainly not deliberative. Deliberative cognitive systems would be conscious, but cognitive systems in general are unconscious. I am not denying the distinction between deliberative and nondeliberative processes. I am just suggesting that it is misleading to suggest that one is cognitive and the other is not; they are both cognitive and reflect the machinations of diverse kinds of neural systems. I would change the focus of inquiry toward understanding diverse forms of information processing in the brain, many of which subserve the organization of action.

BASAL GANGLIA AND THE ORGANIZATION OF ACTION

From the point of view of evolution and behavioral adaptation, the organization of thought is embedded in the organization of action. As early as 1896, for example, Dewey noted in his critique of the reflex arc that cognitive systems are pervasive in the organization of action (see also Prinz, 2003). A number of neural scientists echo this thought in their considerations of the neural circuits; the buildup of behavioral units orchestrated within syntactical systems within the basal ganglia, cerebellum, and motor cortex are now somewhat understood (Graybiel, 2001; Graybiel et al., 1994; O'Donnell, 1999).

Syntactical competence is a form of motor control. In his article on the serial order of behavior, Lashley (1951) extended the language of syntax to basic motor control, opening the context for the cognitive presence within basic motor function. Lashley suggested that syntactical organization underlies the organization of diverse behaviors, not just language.

Central control of motor programs predominates (e.g., Fentress, 1982; Lashley, 1951); deafferented animals are competent in the expression of diverse forms of motor programs, but just as dry mouth is an important signal, so is proprioceptive feedback. The rules (syntax) for the basic units of expression are centrally orchestrated. This is what Lashley and, later, many other investigators called attention to (Berridge & Whitshaw, 1992).

One example of syntactical organization is grooming behavior (Fentress, 1982). The grooming behaviors of several species have been studied for characteristic patterns of behavior. The behaviors are species specific and rule generated (Berridge & Whitshaw, 1992). The behaviors have been studied under diverse conditions. Interestingly, dopaminergic expression can exaggerate the movement sequences and decrease expression of the sequences under conditions of either too much or too little dopaminergic expression (Berridge & Aldridge, 2000; Cromwell, Berridge, Drago, & Levine, 1998). The serial coding of the behavioral expressions is dependent on neo-striatal neurons (Aldridge & Berridge, 1998; Aldridge, Berridge, Herman, & Zimmer, 1993; Fig. 3.4), in which dopamine is an important neurotransmitter for normal behavioral expression. Both too little and too much dopamine reduces competence and options.

Regions of the basal ganglia are linked not to the production of the movements per se, but to the order of the sequences, generating the organized sets of behaviors (Aldridge et al., 1993), and dopamine is one important piece of the neurochemical signature (Fehling, 1966). The organization of thought and the syntactical sequencing of behavior are tied to basal ganglia function (Marsden & Obeso, 1994).

The basal ganglia are involved in a variety of learned behaviors (e.g. Graybiel et al., 1994; Knowlton, Mangels, & Squire, 1996). We know that in diverse species, action sequences are represented in diverse regions of the brain, including the prefrontal cortex. We also know that regions of the basal ganglia, along with Broca's areas and other regions of the frontal/motor cortex, underlie basic syntactical processes (Ullman, 2001; see next section).

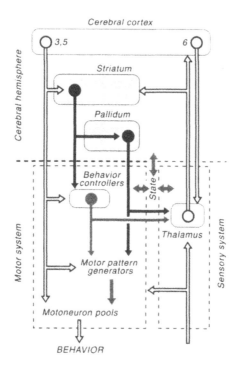

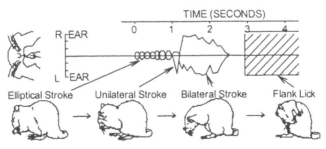

FIG. 3.4. Depiction of the organization of behavior (top, Reprinted from *Brain Research*, 886, L. W. Swanson, Cerebral hemisphere regulation of motivated behavior, 113–164, copyright © 2000, by permission from Elsevier). The syntax phases in grooming. The four syntactic phases—elliptical strokes, unilateral strokes, bilateral strokes, and body licking—are schematized in their drawings. The choreography time line has fourpaw movement as distance from the midline (Right–up, Left–down) as a function of time (x-axis, tics = 1 sec) for a typical syntactic chain (left paw represented by line below the axis, right paw represented by line above the axis (bottom, Aldridge & Berridge, 1998, 2002. Copyright © 1998 by the Society for Neuroscience. Reprinted by permission.)

The point I want to emphasize is that the basal ganglia are involved in a wide range of cognitive functions. Because of high concentrations of dopaminergic innervation, this region of the brain is also linked to the motor and cognitive impairments of Parkinson's disease (Marsden & Obeso, 1994; Mochi et al., 2004). One emerging function of regions of the basal ganglia (e.g., striatum) is the prediction of rewards; for example, in human studies, dopamine transmission in the striatum has been linked to the prediction of monetary rewards (Zald et al., 2004). In fact, different parts of the basal ganglia have been linked to different phases in the learning of events. One study in humans, using fMRI to measure brain activity, has found that the ventral striatum in particular is linked to predictions of reward (O'Doherty et al., 2004; Fig. 3.5).

Let's move now to phenomena usually identified with cognitive systems in the brain.

PROCEDURAL AND DECLARATIVE COGNITIVE/MEMORY SYSTEMS: CORTEX AND BASAL GANGLIA

There are a number of memory systems in the brain (e.g., Eichenbaum & Cohen, 2000; Schacter, 1996), but two stand out. One is procedural memory, and the other is declarative

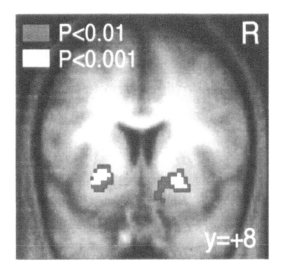

FIG. 3.5. Ventral striatal activation (fMRI) following prediction error signals during Pavlovian conditioning. Reprinted with permission from O'Doherty et al, 2004. Copyright © 2004 AAAS.

memory (Squire et al., 1993). One system has been linked to procedures, rules, and syntax (skills), the other to semantic memory systems. One system has been tightly linked to the frontal cortex and more recently the basal ganglia, the other to the temporal and parietal lobes (e.g., Martin et al., 1996; Ullman, 2004).

Perhaps mistakenly, declarative statements or memory have been associated with cognitive procedures, whereas procedural memory (such as knowing how to ride a bike) is construed as motor and noncognitive (Squire et al., 1993). I think this is a misleading way to characterize the differences between the two kinds of memory, for both reflect cognitive or information-processing systems. Distinctions like procedural and declarative memory have less to do with whether something is cognitive and more with whether something is habitual or new. Moreover, propositional representations are not just the province (as is often construed) of what is conscious, of what is not habitual. Therefore, memory tasks that require distinguishing what Ryle (1949) called "knowing how" from "knowing that" are not assessing the difference between something that is cognitive and something that is not, but rather something that is automatic and well rehearsed and something that is neither automatic nor well rehearsed (Mishkin & Petri, 1984; Squire et al., 1993). Once something is automatic, perhaps it can be relegated to regions of the brain such as the striatum, regions that we know in mammals underlie motor control and developed habits of action (Graybiel et al., 1991; Rolls & Treves, 1998; Fig. 3.6) and language (Lieberman, 2000; Ullman, 2001). But we also know that regions of the frontal cortex that underlie complex behavioral functions can be automatic.

Under diverse conditions, we also now know that regions of the frontal cortex and striatum underlie the organization of syntactical structure. For example, the detection of verb displacements in a sentence activates brain regions such as Broca's area and regions of the basal ganglia, as demonstrated through the use of brain imaging techniques (Ullman, 2001). These sorts of data suggest that the distinction between motor and cognitive structure is very dubious.

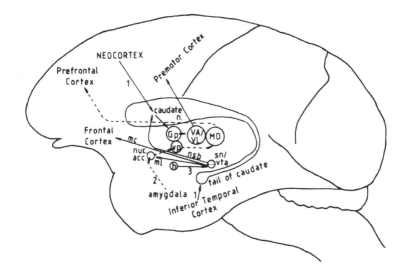

FIG. 3.6. Some of the striatial and connected regions in a lateral view of a macaque monkey brain, upon which is superimposed the activity of single neurons. Gp = globus pallidus; h = hypothalamus; mc = mesocortical dopamine pathway; ml = mesolimbic dopamine pathway; sn = substantia nigra, pars compacts (A9 cell group); nsb = nigrostriatal bundle; nuc acc = nucleus accumbens; vta = ventral tegmental area (adapted from Rolls & Treves, 1998). Reprinted by permission.

An important distinction between procedural and declarative memory is also useful in understanding language and deficits in linguistic expression following neurological damage. This is the distinction between systems that control established motor skills, including the syntactical features of language system (Pinker & Ullman, 2002; Ullman, 2001), from the larger lexical or semantic systems. The distinction was first based on neurological damage (Broca, 1863; Lichtheim, 1885; Wernicke, 1874; see also Pulvermuller, 2002) and then later on a theory of language acquisition (Chomsky, 1965; Pinker, 1994, 1998). Broca's area has been consistently tied to the "motor"components of language (Lichtheim, 1885; Pulvermuller, 2002), in addition to a broad array of information-processing systems including musical syntax (Maess, Koelsch, Gunger, & Friederici,

2001). Although there are many criticisms of this position about language, there does appear to be a distinction between regions of the brain such as frontal cortex (including Broca's area) and the basal ganglia that are tied more to organizing the motor/cognitive functions, and regions of the brain such as the ventral temporal lobe that are tied more to cognitive/semantic or lexical organization (Martin et al., 1996; Ullman & Pierpont, 2005). Both functions are cognitive, so the issue is not whether one is cognitive and the other is not.

Interestingly, parts of the basal ganglia in addition to the frontal cortex have been linked to syntactical organization for human language (Ullman, 2004). Parkinsonian patients have greater impairments with the syntactical features of language than with its lexical components (Ullman, 2001; Fig. 3.7). That is, patients in whom dementia is not an issue still have greater difficulty with the syntactical features of language than with its lexical features, thus reinforcing the distinction between the procedural and declarative features of memory as they pertain to language.

Perhaps it would be more coherent if, instead of referring to cognitive and motor systems when referring, for example, to basal ganglia and frontal cortex involvement in parsing sentences or generating serial grooming sequences, we instead referred to the diverse cognitive systems that underlie motor sequences in behavior; no separation.

PREFRONTAL CORTEX: IMAGINING, WATCHING, AND DOING

Over the past decade, it has become clearer that the basic cortical regions that subserve functions such as vision or audition are active not only when an individual looks at an object or hears a sound, but also when one constructs the seeing (e.g., Decety et al., 1994, 1997, 2002; Frith et al., 1991; Kosslyn, 1994) or hearing through imagination (Kohler et al., 2002). Many of the same neural sites are active in these contexts regardless of whether the context is real or imagined. Of course, this is as it should be: Why should there be an extra imaginative site?

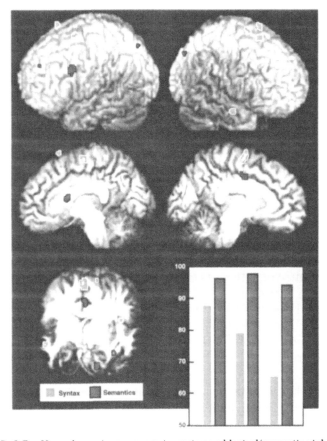

FIG. 3.7. Hemodynamic responses to syntax and lexical/semantic violation detected by fMRI, and the performance (box in corner) of normal (dark) and the percent correct in Parkinson's patients on past-tense production (irregular is on the left, regular is in the center, and the novel verb type is on the right; adapted from Ullman et al., 1997; Ullman, 2001). Reprinted by permission from Nature Reviews Neuroscience, Copyright © 2001, Macmillan Magazines Ltd, and by permission of the author.

Goal objects are represented within the organization of movement and action. Perhaps one of the most interesting findings that has emerged in the study of the organization of action is that there are sets of neurons in the frontal motor cortex that are active when one watches another perform an action and when one performs the same action oneself

(Jeannerod, 1985, 1988, 1994). Cognitive systems in the frontal motor cortex are active when one moves and also when one does not move but rather imagines the movement or watches someone else move (see below).

In fact, at the level of frontal cortex and basal ganglia, representations of goals are endemic to the motor system (what you or I may do). In other words, representations of action are endemic to the motor cortex (Hari et al., 1988; Nelissen et al., 2005; Rizzolatti & Luppino, 2001). One of the most interesting aspects of the motor system's regulation is the cognitive structure that pervades it.

In experiments with macaques, for example (e.g., Rizzolatti et al., 1996; 2000), frontal-motor neurons were active when an animal was shown movement or when it was moving. Thus, grasping for an object or watching another animal grasp the object resulted in the activation of regions of the motor cortex. A storehouse of actions is coded in this region. In humans, researchers have demonstrated that this region is active when an individual watches someone else perform a well-rehearsed, intentional, goal-oriented action and also when the individual performs the action himself (Jeannerod, 1988, 1994).

Other regions of the brain, including the inferior parietal lobe, are active in the representation of action patterns (Gallese, Fadiga, Fogassi, & Rizzolatti, 1996; Perrett, Rolls, & Caan, 1982; Rolls, 1992). Neurons in this region were active both during the viewing of an action and performing the action oneself.

Regions of the temporal lobe are responsive to detection of the direction of a movement made by another, whether or not the movement was intentional. Central representations of the movement are integrated along pathways that are essential in visual and auditory information processing (Kohler et al., 2002; Perrett et al., 1982). Deciphering action by others, in addition to the organization of one's own action, is a fundamental function of the brain, and for visual creatures like humans, the visual cortex plays an expanded role in the organization of action.

The ability to see others in terms of beliefs and desires is an important cognitive adaptation (e.g., Dasser, Ulbaek, &

Premack, 1989) in our evolution and our social knowledge (Baron-Cohen, 1995; Dennett, 1987; Frith & Frith, 1999; Schulkin, 2000; Searle, 1983, 2001). And the neural networks designed to orchestrate the organization of action are recruited when observing and deciphering the actions of others. Diverse cognitive systems are recruited toward the analysis of movement, of goal-intended action (Hari et al., 1988; Jeannerod, 1994; Nichols & Stitch, 2003; Rizzolatti et al., 2000). Regions of the brain are active when one observes another perform an action and when one imitates the action that was just observed (Decety et al., 2002; Fig. 3.8). Early in their development, young children have this ability to easily imitate others and, by doing so, to gather a foothold on the world. The perception of action and the generation of action are recruited

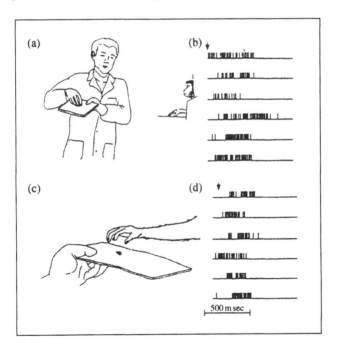

FIG.3.8.   (a and b) Activity of mirror neurons in the prefrontal cortex as a monkey watches an experimenter grasp a food pellet. (c and d) Activity in the same neurons when the monkey grasps the pellet himself (Di Pellegrino et al., 1992: Jacob & Jeannerod, 2003). Reprinted with kind permission of Springer Science and Business Media.

by common cognitive/neural mechanisms that perhaps reflect "ideomotor" regulation (Berthoz, 1996; Deecke, 1996; Freund, 1990; Prinz, 2003). Regions of the brain that underlie action are also recruited in imagination and perception. These neurons are located in regions of the neocortex that underlie behavioral flexibility and greater choice. Not surprisingly then, they are linked to voluntary action. Moreover, the vocabulary of action sequences exists at the level of the frontal cortex, striatum, and cerebellum. Within each of these regions are cognitive/motor systems that underlie the organization of action (Jackson & Decety, 2004).

Evolution and Devolution in the Regulation of Behavior

In the 19th century, Hughlings Jackson and others began to realize that the brain was hierarchically organized, and the more evolved regions of the brain exercised control over the phylogenetically older regions of the brain (Jackson, 1882/1984). Jackson was very much under the influence of Darwin and Herbert Spencer (1855), who coined the phrase "the evolution and dissolution of the nervous system." Evolution is integration, whereas dissolution is disintegration and breakdown.

To Jackson, one form of dissolution that resulted from pathology of the nervous system was epilepsy. First he defined epilepsy in terms of stages, and then he described the pathologic expression and the loss of motor control seen in the disorder. Evolution has to do with the use of motor programs in domains that are more diverse than those for which they were initially selected. Dissolution into epilepsy, per Jackson's example, is the loss of this control, the dissolution of the will.

Jackson (1882/1958) defined epilepsy as a "sudden transitory discharge of some part of the cortex" (p. 9). But Jackson was too enamored of the cortex. The overactivation of regions of the brain, such as the amygdala, that are integral to motivation and its expression in action through the basal ganglia can result in seizure-like responses.

Inappropriate firing of sets of neurons can occur in many regions of the brain, resulting in the loss of voluntary control and organized behavioral sequences. The organization of behavior demonstrates the extent to which the development of sensorimotor function is also a feature in the recovery from brain damage. A classic example is the fact that damage to the lateral hypothalamus or regions of the neocortex in rats and cats results in characteristic behavioral patterns. Such damage results in specific forms of sensory-motor impairments that look very much like the lack of motor ability in the normal neonate. The recovery from brain damage and the return of sensorimotor function looks, to an amazing degree, like the sensorimotor development of these species (Teitelbaum, 1971, 1977). In other words, the pattern of gaining control and flexibility of limbs and the ability to use diverse parts of the body in normal development looks remarkably similar to recovery from extensive damage to several regions of the brain.

Diverse forms of brain damage (devolution of the brain and the organization of action and the expression of the will) interfere with dopamine expression. Consider one example: damage to the lateral hypothalamus. In this case, dopamine levels are reduced by 70% to 80% (Ungerstedt, 1971) and experimentally induced dopamine depletion results in many of the same sensorimotor impairments that result from injury, as well as a recovery process that recapitulates normal sensorimotor development (Teitelbaum, 1971; Teitelbaum, Cheng, & Rozin, 1969). One result is the degradation of motivational competence, expression. One result would be a decrease—as in for example, Parkinson's disease—in the ability to move, to think, to act, to will.

CONCLUSION: NO GHOSTS

There are no ghosts in the machinery of the brain. Strip away the absolute abyss between cognitive and motor systems, and speak in terms of degrees rather than of absolute separation. What is apparent is the degree to which cognitive systems are part of the hardwiring of the motor systems embedded in the brain. Thus, I suggest that a number of cognitive systems in the brain are not separate from the motor programs that underlie behavioral adaptation. Rather, cognitive systems evolved as part of the organization of action (Dewey, 1896; Gallistel, 1992). There is no separation of the motor systems from cognitive systems; there are, I would suggest, just different kinds of information processing in the brain's organization of action. That does not mean that thinking equals doing, or acting. Surely it does not. But only that the evolution of cognitive systems co-evolved with motor systems that underlie willed action.

Disorders of motor/cognitive control, such as Parkinson's disease, represent a loss of motor control and behavioral flexibility and cognitive function (Brown & Marsden, 1998; Cools, 2005). Shaking palsy, such as that seen in Parkinson's, represents a loss of control over voluntary movement and coherent patterns of behavior. Other forms of devolution of motor control are Huntington's chorea and Tourette's syndrome (typified by tics and twitches), genetic disorders in which the genes that regulate dopamine expression have been implicated (e.g., Diaz-Anzaldua et al., 2004).

Regions of the prefrontal cortex and basal ganglia underlie the organization of action, the effectual arm in the serial order of behavior, in the application of rule-governed behavioral options (Aldridge et al., 1993; Fentress, 1982; Lieberman, 2000; Ullman, 2004). Observing others and repeating their actions recruit many of the same circuits in the brain. Perhaps this cognitive capacity plays a role in anticipating the level of effort that the action requires. Underlying the organization of action and thought are neurotransmitters (such as dopamine) and their expression in key regions of the brain. These regions include the basal ganglia and cortical areas, which govern the organization of action. These are the integrative areas of the brain that make possible the action that is essential for adaptation.

4 Self-Control and Behavioral Inhibition

At the heart of our evolution is our ability to carry out diverse goals, achieve successful reproduction, bond with others, develop tools that expand our horizons, and successfully inhibit behaviors until they are timely. This last feature in particular was an essential part of our evolutionary ascent.

Behavioral inhibition is fundamental to self-regulation or self-control. One caveat at the onset: There is more than one sense of behavioral control or inhibition. Behavioral inhibition reflects both reflexive and automatic responses and nonreflexive and less automatic responses. I do not mean to be misleading about behavioral inhibition, for this concept to many people is associated with behavioral flexibility and frontal cortex. And indeed it is (see below). But it need not; behavioral inhibition reflects basic fast reflexes to danger (for example), and more labile systems in which several behavioral options are considered (whether to take this job, buy this stock). Thus, although behavioral inhibition is not the same as neural inhibition, it also does not represent one form of behavior, and reflects both involuntary and voluntary expression. And behavioral inhibition is a cultural value; inhibition and self-control are core values both for Victorians and pragmatists (Smith, 1992).

Thus, in what follows, I discuss several different forms of behavioral inhibition, again suggesting that central dopamine plays an important role. Again, central dopamine expression is just one neurotransmitter among others (e.g., norepinephrine, serotonin, acetycholine), but one in which there is good reason to link it to diverse forms of behavioral expression, including inhibition. But I do not wish to oversell it. Moreover, as I noted in previous chapters, central dopamine is linked to appetitive behaviors, underlying motivational systems in which approach to resources is paramount. In other words, central dopamine expression is neutral with regard to behavioral approach or behavioral inhibition. It is just essential for the organization of action, the organization of information processing in the central nervous system. There is no paradox about why central dopamine expression can subserve both approach and inhibitory behaviors.

BEHAVIORAL INHIBITION

The recognition of the role of diverse regions of the brain in behavioral inhibition has been noted by many investigators in the 19th and 20th centuries, including Jackson, Ferrier, Sherrington, James, and Freud (Finger, 1994, 2000). Simple inhibitory neurons control a wide diversity of behaviors associated with inhibition. Tonic immobility and hypnotic effects in birds in the face of predation is one such adaptive response (Gallup, 1977; Kraines, 1969; Maquet et al., 1999; Rainville et al., 1999).

The origins of behavioral inhibition lie in our biological past, in the ways our brains respond to information and the expression of neurotransmitters fundamental to the organization of action and thought. Several neurotransmitters have been linked to behavioral inhibition (e.g., gamma-aminobutyric acid [GABA], centrally generated dopamine; Kelley, 2004).

Behavioral inhibition is a linguistic term that plays an indexing function in several domains of scientific research. Behavioral inhibition is not the same as an exaggerated sense of fear. Moreover, different tools for measuring inhibition vary across subject matter (Pliszka et al., 2000; Williams et al., 1999). There is more than one meaning of behavioral inhibition. And I will liberally expand the concept to include both reflexes (freezing in fear, social withdrawal) to clear control over behavior. Dewey (1896) identified behavioral inhibition with the origins of emotional struggle, adaptation, and adjustment through intelligent action. He reasoned that inhibition of normal action forces attention to something problematic for which a new solution is needed. This is the view of inhibition that places it under one's voluntary control. But behavioral inhibition is a much broader term. On a continuum that goes from the reflexive (freezing to a snake) to self-regulation (inhibiting a behavior, e.g., ingestion at a water hole to avoid being eaten by a predator), the concept of behavioral inhibition runs a wide semantic terrain.

Indeed, multiple systems in the brain underlie behavioral inhibition. One well-known neural/behavioral circuit is the "freezing" reflex to perceived danger (Fanselow, 1994). This circuit includes regions of the amygdala and frontal cortex in addition to brain stem sites (see LeDoux, 1996, 2000; Pfaff, 1999). Through amygdala activation, diverse regions of the brain are recruited into functional significance. These include the lower brain stem that underlies freezing, the lateral hypothalamus in the regulation of blood pressure, the paraventricular nucleus of the hypothalamus, and the activation of the hypothalamic pituitary axis (Kapp et al., 1979; LeDoux, 1996, 2000).

Looking at a snake can provoke a number of responses, but one response that competes among others is freezing. Fear is not identical to the freezing circuitry in the brain (Kagan & Schulkin, 1995). The circuitry in the brain that elicits the freezing response does not necessarily elicit fear. But the amygdala is one critical region of the forebrain among others that is essential in the perception of danger (Calder et al., 2004; Fanselow, 1994; Gray, 1991; LeDoux, 1996; Rosen & Schulkin, 2004; Weiskrantz, 1956; Fig. 4.1).

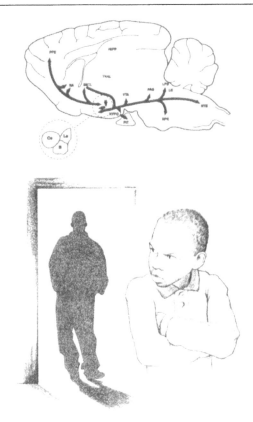

FIG. 4.1.   Fear. Top: Schematic drawing of a neuroamatomical circuit of fear. Major areas and pathways are described but not all are included. The amygdala (circle with the lateral [La], basal [B], and central [Ce] nuclei labeled) plays a central role in the circuit. The lateral nucleus receives most sensory input via the thalamus (THAL) and cortex. The basal nucleus receives input from the lateral nucleus, hippocampus (HIPP), and cortex. The basal nucleus also sends efferents to the lateral portion of the bed nucleus of the stria terminalis (BSTL), nucleus accumbens (NA), and prefrontal cortex (PFC). The central nucleus receives input form the lateral and basal nuclei and has extensive output to diencephelon, midbrain, and brainstem. This includes the hypothalamus (HYPO), ventral tegmental area (VTA), periaqueductal gray (PAG), lateral parabrachial nucleus (PB), locus ceureleus (LC), reticularis pontis caudalis (RPC), and the nucleus of the solitary tract (NTS). As can be seen, many of these areas send reciprocal connections to the amygdala. Major inputs discussed in the text are the prefrontal cortex, nucleus of the solitary tract, and the locus ceureleus (Rosen & Schulkin, 2004). Bottom: A depiction of the fear/anger of a stranger in a child.

Dopaminergić activations modulate amygdala function in a variety of contexts (e.g., Fried et al., 2001; Tessitore et al., 2002). Genetic variance in dopamine production in humans alters amygdala activity in the perception of fear-related objects (Drabant et al., 2004). The perception of a fearful face (for example) activates the amygdala and is compromised under conditions of pathology. Thus, patients with Parkinson's disease have decreased responses (as recorded in the brain through fMRI) than normal subjects to detecting diverse facial expressions, including fearful faces. When pharmacologically treated to normalize central dopamine expression, the behavioral response is restored to normal levels in these patients (Tessitore et al., 2002; Fig. 4.2). Thus, the perception of the snake, just like freezing, requires the activation of dopamine in the brain.

PREFRONTAL CORTEX AND THE INHIBITION OF BEHAVIOR

There is quite a long tradition of associating the prefrontal cortex with the regulation and control of inhibition. It is found in the works of diverse 19th-century neurologists such as

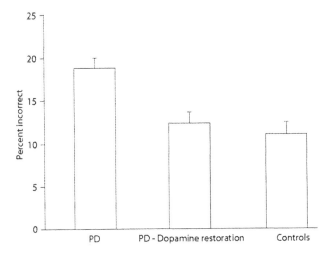

FIG. 4.2.   Percent incorrect responses in a perceptual detection test in Parkinson's patients (PD), patients who have restored dopamine, and in controls (adapted from Tessitore et al., 2002). Copyright © 2002 by the Society for Neuroscience. Reprinted by permission.

Jackson (1882/1958) and James (1890/1952), and it found full expression in the work of Pavlov. Pavlov (1927), like others, was interested in the inhibitory and excitatory mechanisms that underlie the organization of behavior. Pavlov was, of course, interested in "conditional inhibition" and understood that "cortical elements enter sooner or later into an inhibitory state" (p. 251; see also Konorski, 1967; Todes, 2002).

The idea that the frontal cortex played some special role in the inhibition of behavior is found in many areas of the behavioral neuroscience literature. One feature that has emerged is that frontal damage generally results in the overactivation of behavior (Damasio, 1994; Goldstein, 1939, 1944; Luria, 1966). Richter and Hawkes (1939) noted that frontal-damaged animals generated more general activity than normal individuals. Many studies have long linked the frontal cortex and dopamine expression to the regulation of the plans and goals that underlie the inhibition of behavior (Fuster, 1997, 2001; Goldman et al., 1970; Goldman & Nauta, 1977; Goldman-Rakic, 1999; Iversen & Mishkin, 1970; Petrides & Pandya, 1999; Roberts & Wallis, 2000; Fig. 4.3)

Thus, one feature of prefrontal cortex damage is impairment of the ability to inhibit behavior; this, of course, reflects our view of the role of the prefrontal cortex (described later in the chapter) in the development of inhibition (Cummings, 1993; Garavan et al., 1999; Horsley, 1909; Kallio et al., 2001). Diverse studies in rodents have found that damage to the frontal region results in perseveration of conditioned fear related responses; rats with damage to the ventromedial portion of this region were more likely to demonstrate exaggerated fear-related responses during trials in which extinction (learning not to fear something) would normally begin to emerge (Morgan & LeDoux, 1995; Morgan, Schulkin, & LeDoux, 2003; see also Myers & Davis, 2002; Quirk et al., 2000). There is greater dopaminergic activity in the medial prefrontal cortex during diverse events, including those related to fear (Morrow et al., et al., 1999). In other words, interference with dopamine transmission disrupts memory of

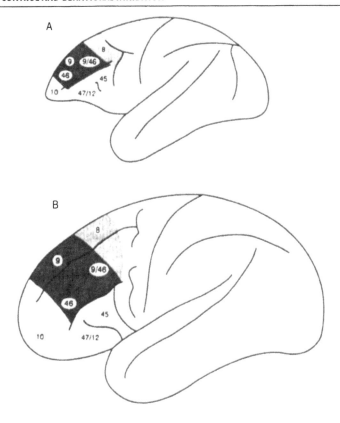

FIG. 4.3.   The mid-dorsolateral (areas 9, 49, 9/46) and mid-ventrolateral (areas 45, 47/12) regions of the frontal cortex in (a) macaque monkey and (b) human brains. From Petrides & Pandya, 1999, Copyright © 1999. Reprinted by permission of Blackwell.

fearful events (e.g., Espejo, 2003; Pezze, Bast, & Feldon, 2003; Fig. 4.4).

A loss of inhibitory control is a feature of prefrontal dysfunction, and more generally this massive area of the brain is linked to diverse cognitive specific and quite general functions (e.g., Damasio, 1994; Denny-Brown, 1951; Fulton, 1949; Fuster, 1997; Goldstein, 1944; Konishi et al., 1999; Luria, 1976; Milner, 1982; Pribram, 1969), to which we will now turn and consider several studies in humans.

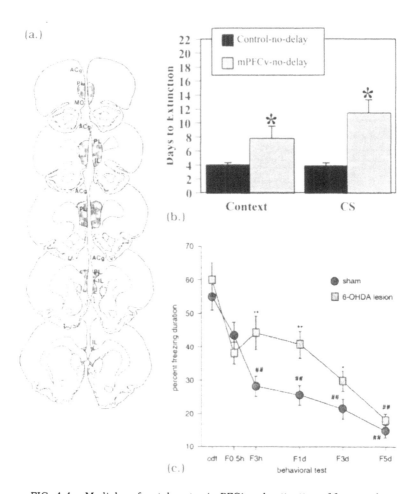

FIG. 4.4. Medial prefrontal cortex (mPFC) and extinction of fear conditioning. (a) Lesion size. (b). Animals with lesions of mPFC take significantly longer to extinguish the freezing response. (c) Rats with dopamine loss in the mPFC display levels of freezing similar to controls during conditioning and during a test 30 min later, but show elevated freezing on tests given 3 hrs, 1 day, and 3 days after conditioning. ((a) and (b) reprinted from *Behavioral Brain Research*, *156*, M. A. Morgan, J. Schulkin, & J. E. LeDoux, Ventral Medial Prefrontal Cortex to the acquisiton and extinction of conditioned fear, 121–130, copyright © 2003, with permission from Elsevier. (c) reprinted from *Neuropsychopharmacology*, *28*, E. F. Espejo, Prefontocortical dopamine loss in rats delays long term extinction in contextual conditioned fear, and reduces social interaction without affecting short-term social interaction memory, 490–498, copyright © 2003, with permission from Nature Publishing Group.)

TEMPERAMENT: BEHAVIORAL ACTIVITY AND CHILDREN

Perhaps more than anyone in the last part of the 20th century, Jerome Kagan has gone to great lengths to describe behavioral inhibition in children and how temperament underlies behavioral inhibition through biological disposition. One way to characterize temperamental differences is by depicting groups of children in terms of those who are highly reactive to strangers and those who are not. Two features of the environment are paramount: the salience of an event and its unfamiliarity. Reactivity is the primary dependent measure. This classification offers a number of predictions (heart rate, cortisol and dopamine levels, and other behavioral and physiological measures). In Kagan's studies, children who were more reactive physiologically were also more sensitive to criticism, shy with peers, timid with regard to danger, and less at ease with adults, all features of behavioral inhibition (Kagan, 1999; Kagan et al., 1988). These temperamental traits are displayed early on in children's development and appear to be genetically based.

Temperamental characteristics pervade behavioral approach and avoidance, the perception of events, and the organization of action (Kagan, 1999; Schmidt et al., 1997). Temperament is part of the explanation for why some individuals are more reactive than others. Shy individuals are socially afraid in unfamiliar contexts.

One example of behavioral inhibition is the wariness to strangers observed in young children. Learning what is safe is one of the most salient characteristics in normal development. Strangers are a source of danger. They are to be approached warily. This is a behavioral adaptation, in which behavioral inhibition is essential to survival. A lack of inhibition can be costly, as can too much inhibition.

Regions of the left frontal cortex are associated with approach behaviors, whereas regions of the right frontal cortex are associated with withdrawal (Davidson et al., 1990; Davidson & Rickman, 1999; Schmidt et al., 1997). Positive stimuli are associated with greater relative activation of the left frontal cortex, whereas negative stimuli are associated with greater relative activation of the right hemisphere (Davidson & Rickman, 1999).

Temperament is reflected in this neural pattern. Excessive inhibition is correlated with greater activation of the right prefrontal cortex and greater avoidance behaviors. Importantly, these phenomena are demonstrable early on in ontogeny (Schmidt et al., 1997).

Subcortical structures, such as the amygdala, are also linked to behavioral inhibition and social wariness. Excessive shyness, or behavioral inhibition in social situations in young children who also had greater cortisol levels, has been shown to lend itself to greater activation of the amygdala when these same subjects were tested later in life (as young adults). When subjects were shown novel and familiar faces, fMRI revealed that those individuals who were described as being shy as children were more likely than normal control subjects to show greater activation in the amygdala in response to the unfamiliar or novel faces. In other words, children described as behaviorally inhibited had greater activation in the amygdala when tested as young adults (Schwartz, Wright, Shin, Kagan, & Rauch, 2003; Fig. 4.5).

Social wariness is an important adaptation, but when it results in exaggerated behavioral inhibition it results in less flexibility and fewer options. Social phobia can be a debilitating and paralyzing disorder that can result in an inflexible outlook and restricted behavioral pattern. Flexibility is one feature of our sense of the healthy child and individual (Daugherty et al., 1993; Milner et al., 1991).

THE DORSAL FRONTAL CORTEX, DOPAMINE, AND BEHAVIORAL INHIBITION

Dopamine receptors are located in diverse regions of the brain, including the prefrontal cortex (Goldman-Rakic, 1999; Goldman-Rakic et al., 1989; Wang et al., 2004), where they also interact with other neuronal signaling systems (e.g., GABA; Mrzljak et al., 1996). The prefrontal cortex is the most heavily innervated dopaminergic region in the neocortex (Bjorkland, Divac, & Lindvall, 1978; Bjorklund & Lindvall,

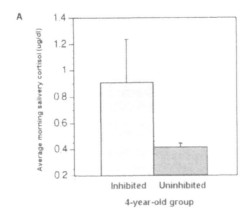

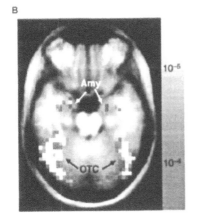

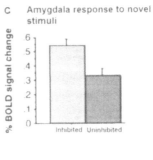

FIG. 4.5.   Levels of cortisol in shy/inhibited children (Schmidt et al., 1997), activation of the amygdala and cortical areas (fMRI) in inhibited in young adults who were diagnosed as children as inhibited (Schwartz et al., 2003). Reprinted by permission from AAAS. Copyright © 2003.

1984) and interacts with pyramidal neurons (Fuster, 1997, 2001; Goldman-Rakic et al., 1989; Fig. 4.6).

Prefrontal cortex and the dopamine receptors in this region (Williams & Goldman-Rakic, 1995) are involved in diverse cognitive functions, including memory (see also Luria, 1966; Passingham, 1975, 1993). Many of the cognitive adaptations that underlie our ability to solve problems in diverse and

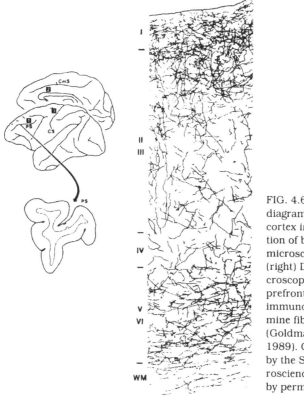

FIG. 4.6. (left) Brain diagram of macaque cortex indicating location of block taken for microscopic analysis. (right) Drawing of microscopic analysis of prefrontal cortex and immunoreactive dopamine fibers (Goldman-Rakic et al., 1989). Copyright 1989 by the Society for Neuroscience. Reprinted by permission.

novel ways have been linked to the prefrontal cortex. It has for years been linked to behavioral regulation, particularly coding behavioral inhibition and memory tasks, which is essential in the ontogeny of behavior and its aberrations following neural degenerative states (Goldman-Rakic, 1987, 1990). Although other regions of the brain are also involved in problem solving, the massive amount of learning that takes place during development requires the prefrontal cortex, which underlies our ability to choose and inhibit behaviors and to delay our responses (Diamond, 2001), skills that are so essential to behavioral flexibility and to exercising our will.

Children born with phenylketonuria (PKU), a metabolic disorder due to a genetic defect, have a disruption in the normal balance of amino acids, a balance which is necessary for the production of adequate amounts of dopamine. These children show impairments in diverse forms of behavioral inhibition (Brunner et al., 1983; Diamond, 2001; Diamond et al., 1997; Pennington et al., 1985; Smith et al., 1996; Table 4.1). Tyrosine is low in these children in relation to the amino acid phenylalanine (Phe). This imbalance can be controlled by dietary means. It was reported early on that dietary regulation, specifically, reduction of Phe intake, can reduce some of the behavioral symptoms in these children. The relative contribution of the two amino acids has been hypothesized to result in a reduced level of tyrosine transport to the brain for the production of dopamine neurons. Now one should note that other systems, including other neurotransmitters, neuropeptides and peripheral hormones are also dysregulated and disrupted by this disorder. Dopamine is therefore just one neural system among others, but it is an important one.

In animal models, this imbalance has resulted in deficits in delayed alternation tests and reduced levels of dopamine in the prefrontal cortex (Diamond, 2001). The major idea is that the dorsal lateral prefrontal cortex is essential for inhibiting responses that disrupt the organization of thought and action. Inhibiting extraneous thoughts is vital.

Human infants and infant and adult macaques, for example, with damage to the dorsal lateral prefrontal cortex are impaired on what is called the A-not-B delayed responses task (Diamond & Goldman-Rakic, 1989; Piaget, 1952; Fig. 4.7). Comparable damage to the parietal cortex did not result in this impairment in behavioral inhibition and the expectation of reward. In other words, behavioral inhibition, in part, requires neocortical development through dopaminergic innervation and expression in the prefrontal cortex.

Children with this amino acid imbalance are impaired on tests of sustained attention and flexibility of thought. This imbalance in amino acid and dopamine has been hypothesized to reflect loss of dopamine synthesis in the prefrontal cortical region (Diamond et al., 1997). This was found across the diverse tasks administered and was independent of the age of the children. Loss of flexibility is the converse of

TABLE 4.1 **PKU Imbalance (Diamond, 2001)**

Mutation in the phenylalanine hydroxylase gene on chromosome 12
↓

Phenylalanine (Phe) is not converted to tyrosine (the precursor to dopamine)
↓

Levels of Phe in the bloodstream skyrocket, while levels of tyrosin in the bloodstream are low

IF PKU *IS NOT* TREATED BY A DIET LOW IN Phe	IF PKU *IS* TREATED BY A DIET LOW IN Phe
The ratio of Phe to tyrosine in the bloodstream is huge ↓	The ratio of Phe to tyrosine in the bloodstream is closer to normal ↓
Widespread brain damage results	Widespread brain damage and mental retardation are averted
Severe mental retardation results	
	HOWEVER
	Blood Phe levels are modestly elevated, and blood tyrosine levels are modestly reduced. Hence: The ratio of Phe to tyrosine in the bloodstream is modestly increased.
	The amount of tyrosine reaching the brain is modestly reduced (because Phe and tyrosine compete to cross the blood-brain barrier).
	Dopamine levels in the prefrontal cortex (but not elsewhere in the brain) are reduced if the Phe:tyrosine ratio in the bloodstream is greater than roughly 8:1 and less than roughly 15:1.
	(Most dopamine systems in the brain are insensitive to small changes in levels of tyrosine. However, the dopamine neurons that project to the prefrontal cortex are different in that they are acutely sensitive to even small changes in tyrosine levels. This is .because these neurons have a higher baseline rate of firing and a higher rate of dopamine turnover. Hence, if the level of tyrosine reaching the brain is modestly reduced, dopamine levels in the prefrontal cortex, but not elsewhere in the brain, are also reduced.)
	Cognitive functions that are dependent on the prefrontal cortex (but not those dependent on other neural systems) therefore suffer.

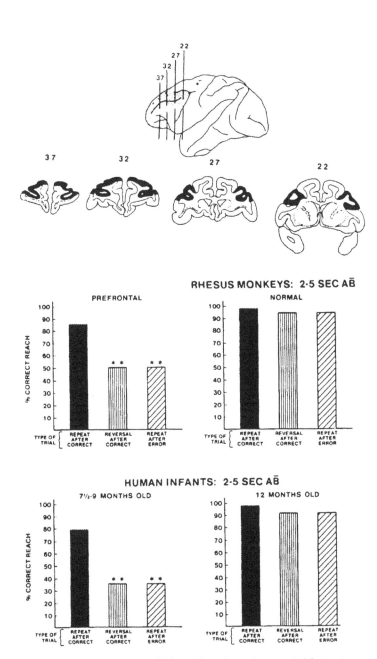

FIG. 4.7. (top) Depiction of bilateral prefrontal cortical ablation in macaques. (middle) Performance of Rhesus monkeys with (left) and without (right) brain damage and of human infants (bottom) on an "A not B" task (Diamond & Goldman-Rakic, 1989). Reprinted by kind permission of Springer Science and Business Media.

our evolutionary ascent (Jackson, 1882/1958), along with the attendant degradation of behavioral options, choice, and the ability to sustain our choices. In a longitudinal study tracing children under various metabolic conditions and testing them for a number of cognitive tasks reflecting activation of the dorsal prefrontal cortex, Diamond et al. (1997) found that treatment restoring the balance of the amino acid tyrosine (to be converted to dopamine) in the brain restored normal cognitive functions. Consider one task in particular: a delayed matching task (Piaget, 1952). This task requires responses that are linked to the prefrontal cortex and that are indicative of behavioral inhibition. This reflects effort and an act of will.

Cognitive functions and behavioral inhibition are altered and restored in some fashion by restoring PKU levels to normal. Both working memory and inhibitory control require the use of the neurotransmitter dopamine in the organization of both thought and action. That is, the key finding from this research indicates that dopamine is the important link between cognitive tasks of working memory and the expression of behavioral inhibition. Amazingly, this metabolic disorder involving an amino acid imbalance can be treated and the behavioral and cognitive impairments thwarted in expression. The results highlight the role of dopamine in the organization of thought, problem solving, and action.

The broad-based molecule dopamine is, thus, essential in the organization of behavior. The range of its effects is quite striking, from a variety of forms of syntactical expression to basic organization of movement and self-control. Indeed, the organization of thought is embodied in the organization of action. It might at first glance seem contradictory for central dopamine expression to be essential for both behavioral inhibition and for the generation or activation of behavior (e.g., expectations of reward; Schultz, 2002). Thus, in this context there are good reasons for dopamine expression playing an important role in the inhibition of behavior. But elsewhere in the brain (e.g., amygdala), dopamine is knotted to the activation of diverse appetitive behaviors. This is no contradiction, since dopamine is fundamental for the organization of action, of which behavioral inhibition is one set of behaviors among others.

HYPERACTIVE CHILDREN

Children with this disorder exhibit a broad array of behavioral symptoms and compromised cognitive functions in multiple settings (e.g., Jennings et al., 1997). These manifest in persistent patterns of inattention and/or hyperactivity-impulsivity. The prevalence of attention deficit/hyperactivity disorder (ADHD) is estimated at 3% to 5% in school-age children. The disorder is much more frequent in males than in females; male-to-female ratios range from 4:1 to 9:1, depending on the setting. In comparison to boys with ADHD, girls with the disorder have lower levels of hyperactivity, inattention, and impulsivity (Oosterlaan et al., 1998; Rubia et al., 1984, 1999; Schachar et al., 1995, 2000).

One plausible view of the ADHD diagnosis is that it reflects the loss of inhibition control.

Some of the behavioral features are depicted in Table 4.2. They include impairments in focus, attention, cognitive competence, and the ability to control one's actions. Thus is the fundamental link between cognitive systems and motor expression revealed in children diagnosed with ADHD.

A number of these aberrations are linked, in part, to a disruption of the dopaminergic systems in the brain. For example, dysregulation of several dopamine transmitter genes has been linked to attentional deficit disorders (e.g., Kirley, 2002; Schmidt et al., 2001). Diverse gene products have been found to affect attention deficit disorders (e.g., Misener et al., 2004; Stein et al., 2005). In a set of diverse studies, the dopamine transporter gene (DAT) was tagged in humans. Brain imaging (e.g., single photon emitted computed tomography [SPECT]) was used on subjects with known attention deficit disorder; what routinely was found to occur was dysregulation of the frontal cortex and striatum (Krause et al., 2003).

On the basis of animal studies, we also know that diverse disease states (hypertension, excessive cocaine consumption; Kreek et al., 2005) may facilitate the onset of attention deficit

TABLE 4.2   **Diagnostic Criteria for ADHD (modified from the DSM–IV)**

Either (1) or (2):

(1) Inattention

    a. Fails to give close attention to details or makes careless mistakes

    b. Has difficulty sustaining attention in tasks or activities

    c. Does not seem to listen when spoken to directly

    d. Does not follow through on instructions

    e. Has difficulty organizing tasks

    f. Avoids tasks that require sustained mental effort

    g. Loses things necessary for tasks

    h. Is easily distracted

    i. Is forgetful in daily activities

(2) Hyperactivity

    a. Fidgets with hands or feet

    b. Leaves seat in situations in which remaining seated is expected

    c. Runs around excessively in inappropriate situations

    d. Experiences difficulty playing or engaging in leisure activities quietly

    e. Is often "on the go"

    f. Talks excessively

Impulsivity

    g. Blurts out answers before questions have been completed

    h. Has difficulty waiting turn

    i. Often interrupts or intrudes on others

disorders. Altered levels of central dopamine expression is one neural/chemical signature that underlies increased salience, hyperactivity, and the breakdown of cognitive/motor adaptations. One result is the breakdown of the will.

CONCLUSION

Behavioral inhibition is a fundamental feature of our evolution and is essential in our ontogeny. Behavioral inhibition is expressed from basic reflexive responses to the choices that we make amid the adjudication of options. In some contexts, there is control by cortical mechanisms; in others there is not. Central dopamine is involved in diverse forms of behavioral inhibition (Tobler, Dickinson, & Schultz, 2004) and at inhibitory synapses themselves (Baimoukhametova, Hewitt, Sank, & Bains, 2004). Dopamine does not function in a vacuum; rather, it operates along with other neurotransmitters such as serotonin, norepinephrine, and GABA. It is one, however, that for some time has been linked to the central control of behavior.

Behavioral inhibition is not the same as neural inhibition, and there are several kinds of events which are referred to as "behavioral inhibition" (Macmillan, 1992, 2000). Nevertheless, our ability to persevere in the face of adversity, and to inhibit impulses that would jeopardize our longer term interests, is to be found in the organization of the chemical codes in regions of the brain such as the prefrontal cortex and amygdala. This is neither the end nor the beginning of the story, just an important part.

Inhibitory self-control is at the heart of our ontogenetic development (Logan et al., 1997; Luetkenhaus & Bullock, 1991). The aberration of this ability for self-regulation and behavioral inhibition is reflected by a number of pathologies, reflecting differences in neural regulation and dopamine expression. Evolution favored our ability not only to run, but to sit, to wait, and to think. The ability to link cognitive control across the range of options is a core feature of humans and is bound to a consideration of our ability to sustain our actions relative to our principles. The expression of motor development and cognitive development are "fundamentally intertwined" (Diamond, 2001). And regions of the brain are specialized to cope with conflict situations (go/no-go experimental paradigm) that reflect choices and with the inhibition of responses.

The sense of inhibition is also a cultural ideal, with self-regulation as a normative behavioral goal; to master our expressions is a deep-rooted value in the Western world, and has its own cultural evolution as an ideal that varies with history (Smith, 1992). Inhibition perhaps is a more primitive term than the concept of the will. But inhibition is complicated and has diverse meanings. Inhibition, as with motivation in the previous chapter, requires effort and something we have called "willpower," and cortical regulation lies at the heart of willpower (Bechara, 2005; Price, 2005).

5 Afflictions

In his great treatise on ethics, Aristotle describes the concept of "incontinence" (from the Greek *akrasia*, literally, "lack of mastery"), a character trait that causes those who possess it to give in to passion, to go against reason and their better judgment in favor of emotion and feeling. The incontinent man, as Aristotle notes, tends to give up, to not persevere—to lack effort and will. Further, Aristotle suggests that the incontinent person is aware of his failing, a breakdown of the exercise of the will). Aristotle is keen to depict the development of the right sorts of habits, the development of the right sorts of commitments, a task rendered easier for someone with the right kinds of disposition, or temperament: "Knowledge must be worked in the living texture of the mind" (*Ethics*, 1974, p. 200).

The addict is a good example. Caught between the habits which now dominate and have raped his capacity to choose what is best for his longer term goals and trying to resist the temptation (e.g., a drug) that now dominates the waking hours of activity, the addict is reduced to a lower level of existence. Most addicts would prefer not to be addicted; they know that their long-term interests (healthy life) are compromised.

The breakdown of the individual in psychopathology is one of the myriad ways in which we are not in control and demonstrates the diminution of the will that results from neurological pathology (Luria, 1976). This is particularly true of diverse forms of addictive behaviors. These are conditions in which excessive desire takes prominence, the range of incentive cues implodes, and there can be a disproportionate link to the actual experience or reward, which has been linked to excessive dopaminergic expression (Berridge & Robinson, 1998; Kelley, 2004; Robinson & Berridge, 1993). Incentives streak our experience by the advertisements all around us, and wanting is what emerges from inside us; one is like a lure from outside, the other like a nudge from within. Motivational states, as I have indicated in previous chapters, have in many contexts been linked to dopamine regulation (e.g., Laviotte et al., 2002).

A narrow notion of homeostatic regulation which underlies addictions and the regulation of the internal milieu did not traditionally take into account higher order cephalic innervation in the regulation of physiological viability via behavioral means of control (McEwen & Stellar, 1993; Schulkin, 2003; Sterling, 2004). Evolved systems were designed to anticipate events and not just to react to events (Barlow et al., 1992; Moore-Ede, 1986). The central nervous system, through its extended innervation of peripheral tissue, plays a large role in physiological viability via behavioral regulation of the internal milieu, the constant use of reward-related neurons (Koob & LeMoal, 2001, 2005).

Fatigue is one consequence of behavioral/physiological systems tirelessly bound to respond to demands that push it beyond its finite capacity (Rabinbach, 1990; Ribot, 1894). There are two historical features about the will: The will is noticed during conflict, and it is a finite resource. Fatigue is often depicted as an expression when the will is exhausted, like the caretaker coming home from work and then greeting her other important jobs (Fig. 5.1). And in general, neurotransmitters are essential for diverse forms of coping behaviors (Coco & Weiss, 2005)

In what follows, I focus again on neuroscience—in this case, the neuroscience of addiction and drug abuse, the role of dopamine in drug use, the vulnerability to abuse and, in this regard, its putative link to reward (e.g., Bechara, Nader, & van der Kooy, 1998; Koob, 1998; Robinson & Berridge, 1993; Wise, 2002, 2005). The concept of the will in regard to vulnerability to addiction has to do with the resistance to temptation. Addiction is a paradigmatic example of an aberrant will, the loss of control, a drain on behavioral/physiological systems, and also of aberrant central motive states (Koob & LeMoal, 2001). These are states of the brain that are linked to a desire and that result in appetitive behaviors (the search for a desired object or condition) and consummation of that desire (Lashley, 1938).

Hence, in this chapter, I explore some of the neural mechanisms that underlie temptation, long-term considerations, predictions of future rewards, and sustaining goals and their expression (Critchley et al., 2001).

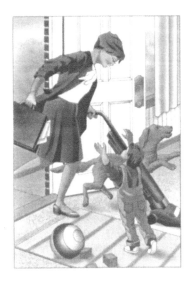

FIG. 5.1.   A modern mother returning home after work.

CENTRAL MOTIVE STATES

Motivational states modulate emotional responses and are inherently tied to information processing (Berridge, 2004; Schulkin, 2003); hence, these states are cognitive (Gallistel, 1992). Central motive states underlie our behavioral responses (Lashley, 1938; Stellar, 1954) and are restrained by our neurobiology. Some of the core features of central motive states are depicted in Table 5.1.

Hormones associated with a particular central motive state prepare the individual to perceive the relevant environmental stimuli that are necessary for obtaining a desired outcome (Schulkin, 2003). For example, the induction of corticotropin releasing hormone (CRH), a neuropeptide, in regions of the brain such as the amygdala and bed nucleus of the stria terminalis, and perhaps the striatum, increases the self-medication from psychotropic drugs (Koob & LeMoal, 2001, 2005). Glucocorticoids are known to increase CRH gene expression in several regions of the brain (Rosen & Schulkin, 2004). Glucocorticoids are known to influence dopamine transmission (Koob & LeMoal, 2001, 2005; Lindley et al., 1999) and CRH is colocalized with dopamine neurons in several regions of the brain. Moreover, elevated levels of glucocorticoids increase dopamine expression and increase the likelihood of diverse forms of self-medication (Piazza & LeMoal, 1997). In other words, elevated levels of this neuropeptide and dopamine and their regulation by glucocorticoids increase the likelihood of self-medication (Di Chiara, 1999; Koob & LeMoal, 2001; Fig. 5.2).

Hormones such as these contribute to approach and avoidance behaviors. These hormones may be mediated through approach and avoidance systems, two primary emotional and motivational circuits in the brain (Davidson et al., 2003; Davidson & Rickman, 1999). There are systems in the brain that generate approach and withdrawal behavior (Davidson, Ekman, Saron, Senulis, & Friesnen, 1990). The appetitive activities of central motive states are mediated by the approach systems (Davidson & Rickman, 1999) through the prefrontal cortex, basal ganglia, amygdala, and hypothalamus. Imaging

TABLE 5.1	**Phases of Central Motive States (adapted from Swanson, 1988)**

Initiation Phase

Deficit signals

Incentive and exteroceptive sensory information

Cognitive information (conditioning, anticipatory)

Circadian influences

Long-term memory

Procurement Phase

Arousal (general)

Foraging behavior

Locomotion

Sensory integration

Previous experience

Short-term or long-term memory

Incentives

Maintenance of viability (visceral integration)

External cues

Consummatory Phase

Programmed motor responses

Discriminatory factors

Satiety mechanisms

Reinforcement

Hedonic motivation

Competition for Behavioral Expression

Multiple motivational states

Environmental factors

Assessment of success/failure

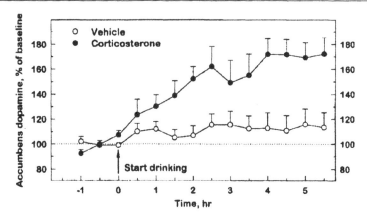

FIG. 5.2.   Ingestion of corticosterone (start drinking) on dopamine levels in the brain region that includes the nucleus accumbens. From Piazza & LeMoal (1997). Reprinted from *Brain Research*, 25, Glucocorticoids as a biological substrate of reward: physiological and pathophysiological implications, 359–372, copyright © 1997, with permission from Elsevier.

and electroencephalographic studies in humans show that appetitive emotions at the cortical level may be lateralized to the left frontal cortex (Davidson et al., 1990, 1999; Schmidt et al., 1997). The left-side of the neocortex is perhaps more closely knotted to approach, appetitive, or goal-directed emotion and not necessarily to "positive" emotion in general.

The basal ganglia, as I have indicated in previous chapters, are important for initiating and terminating movement and for the anticipation of reward (Kelley, 1999, 2004). The prefrontal cortex encompasses two separate and important stages of the approach system. The dorsolateral prefrontal cortex may be important for representation of the goal state in working memory, whereas the medial prefrontal cortex may play a role in retaining the reinforcement contingencies in working memory (Rolls & Treves, 1998). The medial prefrontal cortex also projects to the nucleus accumbens, which is part of the dopaminergic reward system and is discussed in more detail next.

Dopamine in the Brain

As I have indicated, dopamine is widely distributed in the brain. Although dopamine is a major neurotransmitter implicated in the brain's reward system, it is also involved in other regulatory and cognitive systems and in the organization of appetitive motivation and the will. Three primary clusters of dopaminergic cell bodies located in the brain are (a) within the arcuate nucleus of the hypothalamus, which is important for neuroendocrine regulation; (b) within the substantia nigra, important for subcortical movement; and (c) within the ventral tegmental area, important for aspects of reward (Wise, 2002, 2005). From these major cell body clusters, dopamine cells project to numerous areas. The third cluster (the mesocorticolimbic dopamine system) includes the brain system that is important for evaluation of food, drink, drug, social, and other rewards (Berridge & Robinson, 1998). Dopamine projections from the ventral tegmental area terminate in various brain areas, including the nucleus accumbens, stria terminalis, amygdala, prefrontal cortex, anterior cingulate, and limbic areas of the striatum.

Of course, the dopamine reward system does not exist in a vacuum. Neurons in the nucleus accumbens receive input from the hippocampus, brain stem serotonin neurons, and glutamate neurons from the cortex and thalamus. Neurons within the nucleus accumbens contain receptors for many other neurotransmitters (Kelley, 1999, 2004). Destruction of dopamine pathways in animals leads not only to movement deficits but also to failure to work for a reward (Wise, 2002, 2005). Positron emission tomography and magnetic resonance imaging show changes in the dopamine projection sites of the nucleus accumbens, neo-striatum, and prefrontal cortex during various reward activities in humans (Fowler, Volkow, Malison and Gatley, 1999).

The realization that the neurotransmitters for movement and motivation are one and the same led to theoretical links between motivation and muscle. The nucleus accumbens, which lies within the basal ganglia, may be a primary ganglion for the organization of action within the brain. Some time ago, Nauta (1961; Kelley, Domesick, & Nauta, 1982; Nauta & Domesick, 1982) suggested that the nucleus accumbens is an important link between the amygdala and motivation for the organization of action (Mogenson & Huang, 1973). Translation of motivational output from the amygdala to the behavioral outputs of the basal ganglia takes place via the connectivity to the nucleus accumbens (Kelley, 1999; Mogenson, Jones and Yim, 1980; Swanson, 2003). And this is, of course, merely one neural route in the expression of behavioral control.

Sites of Drug Action

Cocaine, an extensively studied drug, has very fast uptake and clearance rates. Its acute effects are mediated by the dopamine system, and the reinforcement and motivation to search for the drug is dependent on the activity of the nucleus accumbens (Graybiel et al., 1990; Koob & LeMoal, 2005; Wise, 2005). Studies with rats show anticipatory neuronal activity in the nucleus accumbens just before lever presses to receive cocaine. Another group of neurons in the nucleus accumbens responds immediately after cocaine infusion, and presumably this activity is directly related to the reinforcing effects of the drug. Injection of a dopamine antagonist directly into the shell of the nucleus accumbens and the central nucleus of the amygdala effectively decreases cocaine self-administration in rats (Caine, Heinrich, Coffin, & Koob, 1995).

Positron emission tomography (PET) imaging studies of human brain activation following cocaine administration show that the nucleus accumbens is one among many areas of increased activation (Breiter, Gollub, Weisskoff et al., 1997). A number of studies have linked elevated dopamine levels with drug reward and craving (Volkow et al., 1997). Dopamine can also be elevated during acute withdrawal (Koob & LeMoal, 2005). Importantly, then, levels of dopamine are altered in both the positive and negative features of addiction. Dopamine is not the neurotransmitter of reward. It is a neurotransmitter essential for the organization of action and thought. Dopamine is involved in the organization and expression of actions, whether positive or negative. Amphetamine administration activates ventral dopaminergic sites and is linked to both the release of cortisol and the subjective ratings of the drug (Oswald et al., 2005).

Many neurotransmitter systems and brain areas are engaged during drug use and abuse. Each drug of abuse involves a different constellation of systems and sites; dopamine is one system involved across the various drug families (e.g., Kish et al., 2001). Animal and human research support the involvement of the frontal cortex in the rewarding aspects of drug use. For example, rats work for cocaine injections administered directly into the medial prefrontal cortex (Carlezon & Wise, 1996). Cue-induced craving in humans addicted to crack cocaine is associated with activation of the left dorsolateral prefrontal cortex (Maas, Lukas, Kaufman et al., 1998) and the orbitofrontal cortex (Grant, London, Newlin et al., 1996); a positive correlation exists between cortex activation and self-reported levels of craving (Maas et al., 1998). Chronic alcoholics who are neurologically normal show metabolic abnormalities in both the medialfrontal cortex and the left dorsolateral prefrontal cortex (Dao-Castellana, Samson, Legault et al., 1998). As I have indicated, there are reciprocal connections between the prefrontal cortex and diverse regions of the basal ganglia (Swanson, 2000, 2003). These two areas of the brain underlie the organization of action and are involved in the planning and carrying out of action. Excitatory (glutaminergic) and inhibitory neurons underlie the behavioral responses (Kelley, 2004).

Changes in the dendrites of the prefrontal cortex are seen in rats receiving prolonged exposure to an addictive substance (Robinson & Kolb, 1997). Drugs of addiction affect cerebral blood flow and glucose metabolism, and the distribution of these changes can give insight into the brain areas that are associated with addiction. Regional cerebral blood flow and glucose metabolism usually return to normal levels after sustained periods of abstinence. Studies in addicted human subjects indicate changes in metabolic activity in orbitofrontal cortex, temporal cortex, cingulate gyrus, and prefrontal cortex (Volkow & Fowler, 2000).

A history of chronic stress interacts with the dopaminergic reward system (Koob & LeMoal, 2005; LeMoal & Koob, 2001). An increase in dopamine release occurs in the frontal cortex of rats exposed to chronic stress, whereas rats without a chronic duress history do not show as much frontal cortex dopamine release when put in the same stressful situation. Chronic duress also leads to a decrease in dopamine in the nucleus accumbens (Koob & LeMoal, 2001, 2005) and to the loss of behavioral control, flexibility, and expression of the will.

Drug Use and Reward

One of the primary reasons for using drugs of abuse is the pleasurable feeling derived from the drug use. However, there are many negative consequences of substance use, and research into addiction attempts to delineate the behavioral and physiological correlates of the components of abuse and dependence.

Pathways to addiction vary between individuals (Koob & LeMoal, 2001, 2005). The drugs' effects are desirable, and motivation for their continued use is dependent on those effects. The negative reinforcement model of addiction states that drug use is the result of a need to alleviate negative states. This self-medication model states that the compulsive nature of drug addiction results from the need for the drug user to feel normal. The self-medication behavior can be triggered by any of a variety of factors, including illness, grief, depression, anxiety, and poverty (Wise, 2002, 2005).

The paraphernalia and social interactions associated with drug use can have a powerful influence on drug addiction beyond the direct effects of the drug itself (Siegel, 1982). Conditioned positive and negative reinforcement are relevant to both continued drug abuse and relapse after prolonged abstinence. If substance use were based purely in unconditioned positive and negative reinforcement (and their underlying neural substrates), then relapse after extended abstinence should not be the social problem that it is in our society. One habit-forming aspect of compulsive drug use is the associative euphoria. The euphoria gets associated with things other than the drug. Examples of conditioned positive reinforcement exist in the animal and human research literature. Animal research suggests that the amygdala and ventral striatum, including the nucleus accumbens, are important for acquiring the conditioned reinforcing effects of stimuli associated with addiction (Everitt & Robbins, 2005; Vanderschuren, Di Chano, & Everitt, 2005). Heroin addicts find injections of saline pleasurable because the conditioned positive reinforcement of the injection is associated with heroin injections and subsequent euphoria. The motivation to continue drug use in order to avoid the negative affective and physiological consequences of withdrawal is a negatively reinforcing aspect of dependence (Koob & LeMoal, 2001). Withdrawal from drug use is associated with decreases levels of dopamine, serotonin, GABA, opioid peptides, neuropeptide Y, but increased levels of CRH and norepinephrine (Koob & LeMoal, 2001, 2005).

Dopamine is important for the craving for drugs, for the salience of associations. For example, a hyper-incentive state plagued by the range of information processing associated with the drug of abuse is mediated, in part, by subcomponents of dopaminergic expression in the central nervous system (Berridge & Robinson, 1998; Kelley, 1999, 2004). We know that one can separate the liking of something (e.g., sucrose) from motor control and intellectual capacity in the struggle to achieve a desired goal. We also know that, for example, in humans, amphetamine infusions increase the extracellular dopamine levels that are linked to both wanting and novelty seeking (Leyton et al., 2002). An overexaggerated set of associations that predominates in the wanting of something, the cognitive resources required to sustain action, and the regulation of motor patterns all require dopaminergic activation. The behavioral responses appear compulsive (Wise, 1987) and the range of associations quite vast in the domain in which dopamine regulation plays a role and underlies the vulnerability to addictive/compulsive expression (Di Chiara, 1999).

Diverse dopaminergic activation in the brain is linked to the desires and incentives of the addicted gambler and drug user. So little reward, so much paraphernalia. The long history of linking dopamine to reward or, for that matter, determining what is rewarding borders on the tautological and nonsensical and has been a source of confusion (Olds, 1955; Olds & Milner, 1954; Wise, 1987, 2005).

The regulation of central dopamine has long been linked to pleasure and, more recently, at the level of the central striatum (Drevets et al., 2001). This connection has been recognized for 40 years in the field of neuroscience. Dopaminergic activation, however, is bi-directional with regard to positive or negative events; dopamine can be activated under both pleasurable and aversive conditions. One of the pleasurable experiences is depicted in Fig.5.3.

The behavioral consequence of introducing dopamine antagonists into the brain/body, which blocks the uptake of dopamine in the brain, is a reduction in the self-administration of amphetamine, cocaine, nicotine, and morphine (Everitt and Robbins, 2005). But there also is a body of literature suggesting that dopamine depletion does not interfere with judg-

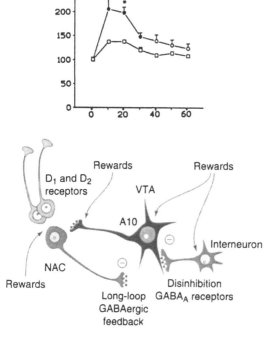

FIG. 5.3. Effect of intravenous cocaine on dopamine in the shell and core of the nucleus accumbens. (Top) Reprinted from *European Journal of Pharmacology, 375,* G. Di Chiara, Drug addiction as dopamine-dependent associative learning, 13–30, copyright © 1999, with permission from Elsevier. And a model of the putative role of dopamine in reward (Bottom) Reprinted from *Trends in Neuroscience, 22,* R. Spanagel & F. Weiss, The dopamine hypothesis of reward: Past and current status, 521–527, copyright © 1999, with permission from Elsevier.

ments about the palatability of diverse objects of consumption (Berridge & Robinson, 1998). In other words, blocking the activity of the dopamine reward system does not axiomatically result in aversion to the food; rather, dopamine antagonists block the craving or desire for the food. The effort to acquire food, and to perform operants, is dramatically decreased after central dopamine depletion.

Animal and human studies assessing the hedonic and incentive responses to dopamine within the reward pathways show interesting results that are relevant to addiction. Dopamine antagonists decrease the desire for a drug. Rats do not self-administer psychoactive drugs when an antagonist is present, but behavioral observation of tongue movements and paw licks show that the rats still "like" the food or drug (Berridge & Robinson, 1998). In contrast, dopamine agonists cause rats to want the drug, but behavioral observation shows that, although the rats are self-administering the drug, they have an aversive reaction, or "dislike," for it. Dopamine is apparently relevant to craving for a drug but not to its hedonic value. A distinction between wanting and liking is evoked; it is possible to want something without liking it, and the mechanisms that underlie these cognitive states appear to be different (Berridge & Robinson, 1998; Robertson et al., 2005). Moreover, excessive dopaminergic expression takes place in response to both desirable and aversive events. Dopaminergic activation occurs in response to both novel events and those that have associative power (cf., Berridge & Robinson, 1998; Horvitz, 2000; Nakahara et al., 2004).

The dopamine pathways involved in wanting are important for the motivational craving experienced by the individual. Whether the individual receives hedonic pleasure from the drug use is no longer important. For most individuals, the hedonic value of the drug is important only during the initial experience of a drug. Once addicted, the appetitive motivational state is concerned only with satisfying the craving induced, in part, by the induction of central dopamine gene expression—an involvement that includes different parts of the basal ganglia, particularly the striatum (Porrino et al., 2004).

Either the overexpression of central dopamine or the underexpression impacts the capacity to link salience of environmental stimuli to predictable rewards (cf., Berridge & Robinson, 1998; Cannon & Palmiter, 2003; Schultz, 2002). For addicts, this reflects the fact that their world is characterized by two major facts. First, once events associated with the drug become salient, they accrue importance astronomically until they dominate and rape the will. Second, over time the pleasure associated with the drug decreases. In other words, the incentive to use the drug grows while the pleasure derived from it decreases (Koob & LeMoal, 2001). Most importantly the addicts' longer term goals are compromised; they can be both hyper-responsive to reward signals and narrow in purview toward their future longer term goals (Bechara, Dolan, & Hines, 2002). "Willpower" requires cortical inhibition of primary areas such as the basal ganglia and amygdala, which underlie our impulsive responses (Bechara, 2005).

Vulnerability to Addiction

A family history of alcoholism is one clear marker of vulnerability to alcohol and drug abuse (Kreek et al., 2005). Studies in adopted and twin children support a genetic risk for alcoholism (Merikangas, 1990). A study by Merikangas, Rounsaville, and Prusoff (1992) stated that 90% of opiate addicts' siblings who experimented with any addictive drug developed a substance abuse problem. The identification of physiological and behavioral markers in those who are genetically vulnerable to addiction can be useful because animal research indicates that environmental factors may induce similar states in those who are not genetically vulnerable. Studies in twins on the genetic and environmental influences on substance use show that genetic vulnerability is more pronounced in men than in women (Jang, Livesley & Vernon, 1997; Van den Bree, Johnson, Neale, & Pickens, 1998). The presence of first- and second-degree alcoholic relatives and multigenerational alcoholism are strongly associated with alcoholism. However, not all children of alcoholics become alcoholics, and not all alcoholics have a family history of alcoholism. For example, one adoption study concluded that the incidence of alcoholism in men with genetic and environmental risk factors of Type I (adult-onset) alcoholism is 11.4%, in contrast to a rate in the general population of about 3.0%; the incidence of alcoholism in men with genetic risk factors of Type II (adolescent-onset) alcoholism was 10.7%, compared with a rate of 2.0% in the general population (Sigvardsson, Bohman, & Cloninger, 1996).

Type II alcoholism is associated with impulsivity and low levels of the neurotransmitter serotonin. Studies of sensation-seeking behavior in children before the onset of pathological behavior and in adults after onset of pathological behavior show a relationship with impulsivity. Although research inconsistently supports the correlative and predictive value of the other dimensions in this theory, the usefulness of the novelty-seeking/impulsivity dimension is upheld consistently (Howard, Kivlahan, & Walker, 1997; Sax & Strakowski, 1998). Evidence from animal research indicates that the relationship between sensation-seeking and impulsivity is probably related to dysfunction of the reward system of the limbic-medial frontal cortex and involves the dopamine circuitry within this system (Di Chiara, 1999; Koob & LeMoal, 2001, 2005).

Novelty-seeking characteristics with early signs of aggressive behavior in childhood appear to be predictive, though not necessarily causal, of pathology in late childhood and adolescence (Masse & Tremblay, 1997). High rates of impulsivity and novelty-seeking behavior in children as young as 6 years, are stable across childhood and are predictive of early alcohol, tobacco, and drug use. Kindergartners who are impulsive and who show little anxiety are much more likely to engage in risk-taking behaviors later in life than children who do not show these two characteristics (Masse & Tremblay, 1997).

High rates of novelty-seeking behaviors exist in individuals with alcoholism and other substance use disorders. These individuals show characteristic signs of "frontal dysfunction" on neuropsychological test batteries (Dao-Castellana et al., 1998). One problem with drawing predictive conclusions from this research is that substance use can have a causal effect on novelty-seeking behavior (Sax & Strakowski, 1998). Also, impulse control problems may contribute to the likelihood of engaging in risk-taking behaviors, such as substance use, without being an explicit cause.

Novelty-seeking has been linked to dopaminergic expression in the brain (Di Chiara, 1999). If such a relationship exists, dopaminergic expression would underlie both an exaggerated sense of seeking reward and, when this sense is exaggerated, an ability to find satisfaction and a tendency for these systems to exhaust themselves (Koob, 1998; Koob & LeMoal, 2001). Amphetamine-induced increases in dopamine are linked to greater novelty-seeking (Leyton et al., 2002). Not surprisingly, some data suggest that Parkinson patients with dopamine dysregulation who are described as having rigid and compulsive cognitive expressions show a decreased response to novel stimuli.

FURTHER EXAMPLES OF THE DISSOLUTION OF THE WILL: ABERRATIONS OF THE BRAIN

In animal studies, environmental events, such as prolonged maternal separation, can result in greater psychomotor activation in response to amphetamine and in greater dysregulation of both central dopamine expression and the hypothalamic-pituitary-adrenal axis (Meaney et al., 2002). In addition, maternal care in rats is associated with dopamine levels; the greater the lick behavior (rats lick their young) the greater the level of central dopamine. The dopamine is actually elevated before the bout of licking behavior, in anticipation of the behavior (Champagne et al., 2004) and more generally perhaps in affiliative bonding (Depue & Morrone-Strupinsky, 2005; Fig. 5.4).

The important point is that the connections that we form with one another are the important ingredient of meaning in our lives (Jaspers, 1913/1997). When in the right context, they can reduce the vulnerability to self-destructive behaviors. This adaptation, for many reasons, is undermined during diverse forms of pathology (Berrios & Gili, 1995).

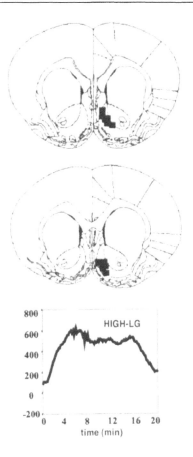

FIG. 5.4. Elevated dopamine before the onset of grooming behavior (adapted from Champagne et al., 2004). Copyright © 2004 by the Society for Neuroscience. Reprinted by permission.

Karl Jaspers (1913/1997), a profound and important investigator of the human condition, understood that volitional acts are tightly bound to drive and impulses and that the will is bound to movement. And diverse forms of pathology are revealed in distorted movements, what he called the "psychotic motor phenomenon" (p. 179). More importantly, he understood something about the isolation that results from diverse forms of human pathology, that disease states of the brain, such as schizophrenia, can entail a recognition of the loss of will, the breakdown of coherent/adaptive action.

Consider two other disorders that reflect the dissolution of the sense of agency fundamental to our notion of the will, and which are related to central dopamine regulation. One should realize that a compromised sense of the will does not reflect one phenomenon, but a range of phenomena; a person with spinal damage cannot move or walk, but expends effort in recovery. The will in this context is not effectual. In other words, the point is that the will is not manifest in action. This, of course, is quite different from the addict who expends effort to procure the drug, but whose long-term interests are compromised. These are still different from the patient with a thought disorder who is unable to get certain thoughts out of their sense of the world and themselves.

Schizophrenia

The characteristic symptoms of schizophrenia include a range of cognitive and emotional dysfunctions that involve perception, inferential thinking, language and communication, behavioral monitoring, affect, fluency and productivity of thought and speech, volition and drive, and attention (Liddle, 1994; Liddle et al., 2001; Pujol et al., 1999; Rapport & Wise, 1988; Robertson & Taylor, 1985; Sawa & Snyder, 2002; Spitzer, 1997; Waldo et al., 1986).

Three features of schizophrenia are linked to the will, as Frith (1992) points out:

1. Limitations in the organization of action
2. Perseveration of expression
3. Involuntary and inappropriate expression

They also include (Heinrichs, 2001):

1. Premature decision making
2. Negative cognitive bias
3. Externalizing attributions
4. Inaccurate speech tracking and monitoring
5. Semantic hyper-priming
6. Impaired theory of mind

Schizophrenia occurs in 0.2% to 2% of the general population. Stereotyped and impaired motor performance is a dominant feature, perseveration of thoughts and movements a common theme (Andreasen et al., 1999; Baker & Morrison, 1998). Alterations in dopamine levels, which may impact both cognitive and motor expression, have long been linked to this pathology. Whatever its etiology, schizophrenia is marked by the features of an inability to control one's thoughts, a compromised sense of agency and ownership, an inability to reduce "noise" that is unrelated to real events, and an inability to anticipate events that are essential in a real context (Posada, Franck, Georgieff, & Jeannerod, 2001).

Schizophrenia is associated with abnormalities of the frontal cortex, which is linked to both working memory and thought disorders (Braver, Barch, & Cohen, 1999; Goldman-Rakic, 1999; Wang et al., 2004; Weinberger, 1988). Altered dopamine levels have been demonstrated in individuals with this disorder (Schatzberg et al., 1985), and links between elevated levels of cortisol and altered dopamine transmission in regions of the brain such as the prefrontal cortex have been suggested (Cohen & Sevan-Schreiber, 1993).

It has been suggested, for some time, that the dysregulation of dopamine in diverse regions of the brain contributes to schizophrenia. A recurring feature of this pathology is the loss of cognitive ability; this includes a degraded ability to filter out information that is not relevant—leading to sensory overload, an exaggerated sense of the salience of events, a reduced ability to demonstrate simple blocking effects, and alterations of prestimulus filtering (screening out information; Swerdlow & Young, 2001), all examples of reduced sensory gating. Sensory-gating alterations are known to be linked to exaggerated dopaminergic function in animal studies (e.g., Schwarzkopf et al., 1992; Swerdlow, 2001), and depletion of central dopamine is known to reverse some of the behavioral impairments (Swerdlow, 2001).

Amphetamine levels exacerbate the symptoms of schizophrenic subjects, in part by altering central dopamine levels. Increased levels of dopamine subtypes are also associated with schizophrenia (Carlson et al., 1997). One view of the etiology of schizophrenia is that the hippocampus, which is known to be tied to declarative memory, might reflect dopamine hyperactivity (Krieckhaus et al., 1992). Other regions of the brain that have been implicated in the etiology of this disorder include the habenula, striatum, and frontal cortex (Goldman-Rakic, 1999). Dopamine, in addition to other neurotransmitters (e.g., serotonin), is very much involved in the etiology of this disorder.

Delusions are a fundamental feature of this condition, and PET studies have linked diverse regions of the brain, including the parietal cortex and cerebellum, to a loss of agency and ownership of one's thoughts and actions (Blakemore, Oakley, & Frith, 2003; Seidman et al., 1995; Spence et al., 1997). The experience of agency is an important part of the concept of the will, and brain regions such as the parietal lobe (Farrer & Frith, 2002), in addition to the frontal and the insular cortex, are critically involved.

Obsessive-Compulsive Disorder

Cognitive expectations guide behavior. Overexpression of the rules guiding behavior generates rigidity, an inability to follow through with the behavior, producing a condition in which one is frozen into a behavioral pattern that is outside of one's will. Obsessive-compulsive disorder (OCD) is characterized by rigid behavioral patterns (Schwartz, 1977). Obsessions, in the form of persistent thoughts, play the role of the "rules," causing distress and anxiety to the individual (e.g., Janet, 1906; Rachman, 1998). Compulsions, the responsive behaviors to the obsessions, are usually repetitive and serve to decrease the anxiety caused by the obsessions. The will becomes immobile as a result of the displacement of normal behavior.

Obsessions and compulsions are comorbid with a number of obsessive disorders, including Tourette's syndrome, trichotillomania, and Orrychophagia (Cohen et al., 1994; Greenberg, 1997; Saxena et al., 2002; Saxena & Rausch, 2000; Swerdlow, 2001). There are genetic vulnerabilities to

OCDs, and there is further comorbidity with depression and anxiety (Baxter & Brody, 1996). The lifetime prevalence of OCD is believed to be approximately 2.5%. Treatment with therapeutic agents that selectively inhibit the reuptake of serotonin decreases some of the behavioral expression of the disorder, including obsessiveness, rigidity, and compulsiveness (Barr et al., 1992; Baxter et al., 1996; Greenberg, 1997; Greenberg et al., 1997, 2000; Hansen et al., 2002; Hollander et al., 1990).

Patients with Tourette's syndrome have a number of behavioral impairments (obsessive behaviors, attention deficit disorders; Eidelberg et al., 1997; Leckman et al., 1995, 1997; LeVasseur et al., 2001). We know from these studies that the basal ganglia are crucially involved in ritualistic behaviors; these are well-formed behaviors that, under pathological conditions, are exaggerated in expression and that perhaps have their roots in fixed behavioral responses seen in more rigidly defined behavioral repertoires in lower animals (Baxter, 2003; Baxter & Brody, 1996; Insel, 1992; Insel et al., 1985; Fig. 5.5).

Indeed, in animal studies, selective lesions of the nucleus accumbens have been shown to result in impulsive behaviors. For example, damage (in rats) to the nucleus accumbens can result in what could be described as impulsive choices. Why? Because rats with such lesions were less able than control rats to choose the better reward when choice was delayed (see Cardinal et al., 2001). And in strains of mice in which dopamine was engineered to be elevated in the brain, there is a greater degree of stereotypic species-specific behavior that looked a lot like that described for obsessive-compulsive or Tourette's syndrome (Berridge et al., 2005).

Regions of the brain such as the basal ganglia are fundamentally involved in the organization of motor control. Perhaps one way in which to envision the basal ganglia is as the head ganglia in executing action and motor control, an integrative area for cognitive/motor systems (Graybiel, 2001; Ullman, 2001). James (1890/1952) noted that the organization of thought and the organization of action recruit many of the same functions. This region of the brain has long been

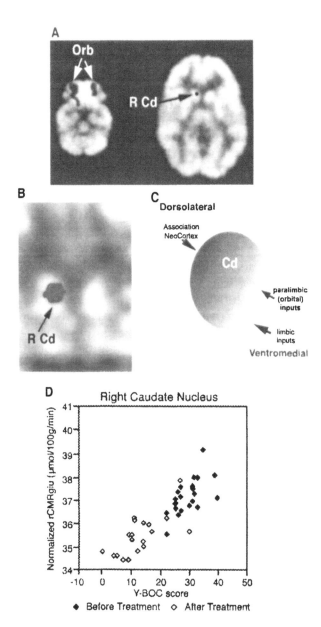

FIG. 5.5. Orbitofrontal cortex and right striatial overactivity in a patient with OCD. (a) PET scan depicting overactivity in OCD patient, (b) particularly in the head of the caudate nucleus (R Cd). (c) Regional projections to Cd. (d) Correlation of right Cd brain activity with OCD symptom severity score. Reprinted from *Physiology and Behavior, 79,* L. R. Baxter, Jr., Copyright © 2003, with permission from Elsevier.

thought to underlie species-specific behavioral responses (MacLean, 1978) and to be anatomically tied to visceral systems that underlie the emotions and motivated behaviors (Heimer, Switzer, & Van Hoesen, 1992; Nauta & Feritag, 1986).

Cephalic programming is at the heart of the organization of action and the everyday habits that are codified in action. The frontal cortex represents a third of the human brain. Interestingly, as I indicated in a previous chapter, we use many of the same motor resources of the brain when we imagine moving and when we actually move, and the motor cortex is fundamental in both cases (Berthoz, 2002; Decety et al., 1997; Jeannerod, 1988; Rizzolatti et al., 1996). Brain imaging studies show activation in diverse regions of the brain, including the prefrontal cortex, cingulate gyrus, and basal ganglia, during real and imagined movement (Fig. 5.6).

CONCLUSION

We know something about the neural mechanisms that underlie compulsive choices, such as those reflective of addictive behaviors. The mechanisms that underlie choice, behavioral control, and vulnerability have an impact on the expression of our afflictions and our vulnerability to addictions of diverse sorts. For several centuries, it has been known that the prefrontal cortex is linked to voluntary action. In common neuroscientific language, this region is vital in the execution of behavior, the assessment of events, and the organization of action (Goldman-Rakic, 1999; Robbins, 1996). The prefrontal cortex is involved in attention, various forms of memory, and sensorimotor integration (Fuster, 2001). The cortical frontal/motor system is what makes the will "real" from an evolutionary point of view (Rizzolatti & Luppino, 2001). The range of functions that involve this region are fundamental to high-level cognitive processes as well as basic motor tasks. Imagery of the planning, perceiving, and execution of intentional action is reflected in the activation of this region of the brain (Castelli, Happe, Frith, & Frith, 2000; Deecke, 1996).

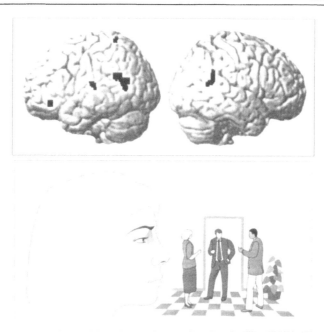

FIG. 5.6.   Thinking about others and activation of the lateral region of the left hemisphere (fMRI) when thinking about imitation. Reprinted from *Neuroimage, 15*, T. Chaminade, A. N. Meltzoff, & J. Decety, Does the end justify the means: A PET exploration of the mechanisms involved in human imitation, 318–328, copyright © 2002, with permission from Elsevier.

One view of the cortex is that it exercises control over the phylogenetically older functional areas in the brain (James, 1890/1952; Jackson, 1882/1958). The cortex pertains to inhibition and behavioral control. However, it is not privileged with regard to cognitive systems; the entire brain is a cognitive machine. Cognitive systems were selected, as were other adaptive systems in the body, and they are endemic to brain function (Grossberg, 2000). Dopamine is a fundamental neurotransmitter that is involved in decision making and the organization and breakdown of action for the expression of the will (Korpi et al., 1987; Shenton et al., 1992). The overactivation or depletion of this transmitter is related to several pathologies that reflect the breakdown of the will, cognition, and viable long-term action.

Failures of the will have long been linked to failures of thought, but in the case I have emphasized, it is also a failure of agency and ownership of one's actions. The extent to which we are able to get our thoughts in line with effort and the will predicts to what degree we have at least a fighting chance of achieving our goals. The addict does not want to live in the ways that are killing him and hurting those around him. He wants not to do it. He desires, he believes, but he looks impotent despite wanting to "just say NO" (to paraphrase Nancy Reagan).

The addict is trying to be free from what he wants. But his whole world is wrapped up in the environments in which he is embedded. The addiction is not just in his head, but also in the massive world of associations. The range of associations can compromise, often does *sabotage*, the longer term goals of reaching sobriety. The issues that surround the cognitive resources are the range of conflicting interests, motivations, and desires. An effective will is reduced. The outcome is the continuation of drug use.

William James, a pragmatically optimistic but beleaguered individual, sought a path of self-mastery and discipline. Part of the meaning of life is in the connections that we have to each other and the bonds that we display (Jaspers, 1913/1997).

We now turn to the rationality of choice.

6 Choice, Control, and the Brain

The brain itself spends a lot of its cognitive resources tagging uncertainty (Schultz, 2002), and probability devices are operative at various levels of the neural axis, including the basal ganglia (e.g., Glimcher, 2003; Knowlton et al., 1996). Some of the cognitive systems are selected by our evolutionary past to adapt to changing circumstances; our evolved brain coupled with a long developmental course amid a rich cultural ambiance, reflects the range of choices and our evolving sense of freedom (Dennett, 2003; Dewey, 1925/1989).

In this chapter, I argue that effort or the will is integral to our ability to maintain long-term goals over short-term satisfaction. Cognitive systems underlie our choices, the control over behavior, and the prediction of events. One rational method of staying the course toward longer term goals (Ainslie, 2001, 2005) is by precommitting ourselves, binding ourselves to future action in order to increase the likelihood of our actually following through (Elster, 1979, 2000). Underlying rational choice is the prediction of future reward outcomes. One neurotransmitter that participates in this process is central dopamine.

Thus, in this chapter, I discuss self-regulation and the expression of effort or the will; a realistic sense of human reason which is important for an understanding of effort and the will; the important role of precommitments to the organization of action, choice, and short and longer term decisions; and, finally, the role of dopamine in the prediction of reward or evaluation of objects.

DEMYTHOLOGIZED HUMAN DECISION MAKING AND ACTION

From a psychobiological perspective, we can say that we are often "good-enough cognitive systems," an idea akin to "good-enough mothering"—just as there is no perfect mother, so too is there no perfect human information-processing system. There is no perch on which to hide in human information processing. Good-enough visceral processing is an essential ingredient of information-processing systems in the mammalian species. The visceral input pervades the processing at many levels of the neural axis and underlies our sense of effort and the will (Swanson, 2003).

In understanding the cognitive mechanisms that underlie the organization of action, and in understanding the will, one must first demythologize human reasoning, highlighting the forms of constraints and biases that pervade decision making (e.g., Baron, 2003; Kahneman, Slovic, & Tversky, 1982; Simon, 1967). Moreover, understanding decision making and its pathology, while demythologizing human reason from the pantheon of perfection to the rough-and-ready tasks to be solved (Kahneman et al., 1982–1989; Simon, 1967, 1979, 1982), is a recognition of a broad array of cognitive orientations that can limit our inferences and decision making, compromise or energize the organization of action and the expression of the will (Ainslie, 2001, 2005).

We are oriented, though this orientation to events competes with others, to assessing utility functions, and one feature in that utility is basic pleasure and pain (Bentham, 1789/1948;

Kahneman, Diener, & Schwartz, 1999). The brain is oriented to compute diverse kinds of utility functions, a predilection to compute and be oriented toward statistical outcome (Glimcher & Rustichini, 2004). These utility functions are not just simple pleasure/pain dimensions, and they are far from perfect. And we are rich in quick heuristic appraisals that organize actions (e.g. Gigerenzer, 2000; Simon, 1982).

A range of biases (Baron, 2003; Kahneman et al., 1982) are inherent in human information-processing systems. Some of the biases are simple heuristic tools for making sense of events. *Bias* is a word with a bad reputation, but to me it is a description of an orientation that we have. Rough-and-ready heuristics underlie human information processing (e.g., Gigerenzer, 2000; Fig. 6.1), and they serve us quite well despite being imperfect. But then, perfection is the very myth about us that should be discarded. When we demythologize human information processing, rationality is downgraded to basic problem solving (Dewey, 1910/1965; Peirce, 1878/1992a, 1878/1992b, 1892/1992c).

In Herbert Simon's terms, instead of perfect rationality, we get "bounded rationality": problem solving in proportion to the problematic context. There are, for the most part, no perfect fits, but, rather, "good-enough" fits that are *satisficing* (see Fig. 6.1), as Simon called it; in more modern terms, heuristics serve adaptation. Rationality, sized to human proportions, generates systems to promote better problem-solving mechanisms (Baron, 2003; Dewey, 1910/1965). Many diverse thinkers have outlined the limitations of perfect rationality (e.g., Elster, 1979; Simon, 1982;

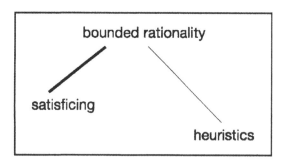

FIG. 6.1. Human information processing. (adapted from Gigerenzer, 2000; Simon, 1982, 1983).

Tversky & Kahneman, 1974). In the context of effort and the will, the acceptance of these limitations are important for behavioral strategies that bind ourselves to certain trajectories, that keep us on track.

Choice: Short- and Long-Term Considerations

An insightful investigator, Ainslie (2001) noticed that "theories almost never mention the will." The breakdown of will is the devolution of behavior in addictions and afflictions that do not reflect rational long-term behavioral expressions and choices. Our ability to restrict choice for future good is at the heart of our precommitments that organize behavior. The goal is to sustain and create behaviors that provide long-term sustenance amid endless short-term seduction.

Ainslie is right to point out that utility theory is about maximizing reward and that we are motivated to do so, but not about the failure of valuing future good in relation to the delay (hyperbolic discount curve). It is the delay of reward, the ability to postpone gratification, the expression of behavioral inhibition, where one important feature of the will reveals itself.

Individuals, despite the claims of classical economic theory, do not always try to maximize their reward. They decide on different types of reward at different rates. This differential discounting is a function of the delay (D). For example, if you offer subjects a choice between receiving $100 tomorrow and $200 in three years, most will choose the $100. In other words, people can and do devalue future rewards proportionately to their delay (Fig. 6.2). Of course, this isn't necessarily flawed, as the probability of actually getting the reward most likely diminishes over delay time. The point is that intertemporal choice is far from being consistent.

Utility theory, like variants of behaviorism, packs a lot into the concept of reward (Rachlin, 2000), one of the most difficult concepts within the behavioral sciences. But the concept of reward is not isomorphic with the concept of pleasure (Ainslie, 1975, 1999; Glickman & Schiff, 1967; Wise, 1987;

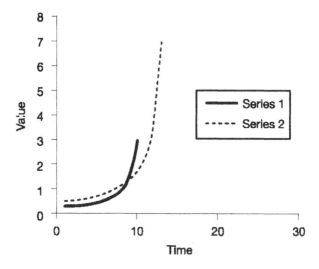

FIG. 6.2.   Hyperbolic discount curves from two rewards of different
sizes available at different times. The smaller reward is temporarily pre-
ferred for a period before it is available, as shown by the portion of its
curve that projects above that from the later, larger reward (Ainslie,
2001). Reprinted by permission.

Wise & Bozarth, 1987; Table 6.1). What Ainslie has noticed is
the competition between reward and pleasure and the various
interests that compete in our internal life, much like the
model of competition in the marketplace. The cyclist balances
her recognition of discomfort with the longer term goal of finishing the race, the reward of finishing (or wining) versus the
discomfort. Reward is a broader concept than sensory
pleasure.

Restricting choices and achieving rationality is to reduce
the seduction of never-ending pulls from the environment
(Chung & Hernstein, 1967). The long-term adaptation of
achieving one's goal means resurrecting paths that are less direct and creating barriers against failure (Hernstein, 1997;
Hernstein & Prelec, 1992). Self-control becomes linked to
self-prediction (cf., Kirby, 1997; Rachlin, 1995, 2000;
Rachlin & Green, 1972; Stevenson, 1986; Thaler & Shefrin,
1981). And self-regulation reflects the rules that one has
adopted to guide and sustain human action. One strategy for

TABLE 6.1   **Zones of Temporary Preference Duration**

Descriptor	Distinguishing feature	Duration of cycle	Time until recognized as problem	Examples
Optimal	Never aversive	None	Never	Conflict-free satisfactions; "to love and to work"
Compulsions	Controlled by willpower; ambivalent feeling of aversion	Months to years	Decades	"Workaholism"; constrictions of personality-like miserliness, anorexia nervosa
Addictions	Clear periods of pleasure and aversion	Hours to days	Days to years	Substance abuse, explosive emotional habits
Itches	Ambiguous pleasurable phase but conscious participation	Seconds	Minutes	Physical itches, obsessions, tics, mannerisms, hypochondria
Pains	Never pleasurable, no participation	Fraction of a second	Fraction of a second	Physical pain, panic

Depiction of Diverse Behavioral Expressions and Their Purported Duration (Source: Ainslie, 2001)

reducing impulsive choices is, by grouping choices together, sets of choices that organize diverse behaviors. Perhaps this might embolden our sense of will power, staying the course for future-related decisions and solidifying a behavioral framework. For the addict, for example, this is an essential cognitive/behavioral adaptation.

But long-term outcomes are uncertain, and short-term gains dominate the experimental literature in animals and people. We are inconsistent, but in some contexts we can focus on a longer term gain and sustain rational action (Loewenstein, 1996, 1999; Loewenstein & Schkade, 1998). Context matters.

As Ainslie (2001) defines the event: "The will is a recursive process that bets the expected value of your future self-control against each of your successive temptations" (p. 89). This is a consideration of the will that is reflected in the context of the organization of thought and action, in which competing resources do battle. Moreover, the competition reflects "a marketplace in the brain" (Ainslie & Monterosso, 2004), and that market place of intertemporal choice activates different brain regions. In an fMRI study, immediate monetary reward choices reflected striatal and limbic regions of the brain, while delaying monetary rewards reflected the frontal cortex (McClure, Laibson, Loewenstein, & Cohen, 2004).

The drama of life is averting the seduction of the omnipresent impulses that undermine our long-term goals (Elster, 2000; Parfit, 1984; Pears, 1985). The will functions in our epistemological lexicon as "a bargaining situation where credibility is power" (Ainslie, 2001, p. 127). The will ensures the credibility of the commitments (e.g., Hirschman, 1981).

Self-control is the desired result. We are working against achieving ends that undermine our long-term interests. But the other side is the vulnerability to excessive control, compulsions, rigidity, and excessive restriction of choice. For those afflicted, this is a reasonable recourse toward mental health. For those to which risk taking is within the bounds of reason, there is more flexibility, because there is more capacity. In other words, part of what we mean by a "healthy will" is based on rational self-control and the development of what James called "soft habits" (see Rachlin, 2000) and the expression of rational goals and their embodiment in worthy habits that we acquire and sustain (James, 1890/1952).These commitments bind our cognitive resources and forms of behavior to forestall some immediate reinforcement.

Of course we often ask whether we could have reasonably made a different choice, not doing what one knows is a better choice (Davidson, 1969; Frankfurt, 1988). Returning to the problem of the addict discussed in chapter 5, "the unwilling addict's will is not free" (Frankfurt, 1988, p.20). Second-order desires, the desires to desire not to do x or to do y, reflect the kind of control that is essential for a healthy will. But perhaps the issue is best expressed not in terms of first- and second-order desires, but rather in terms of diverse conflicting motives and appetites and desires that compete for cognitive and behavioral expression. Those who achieve some measure of freedom line up these conflicting desires with their behavioral expression, which is surely an achievement and a constant challenge. In fact, the capacity to choose not do x is essentially related to efficacy and the expression of the will (Pink, 1996).

Regulating and taming future behavior, precommitting ourselves to behavioral options, is one adaptation to offset the tendency to not stay the course (e.g., Ainslie, 1975; Elster, 1999, 2000; Elster & Skog, 1999). But when it comes to overcoming addictions and afflictions, the ability to stay on a course obviously becomes more difficult to instantiate and make real. Let's turn to "taming chance."

Limiting Choice: An Essential Behavioral Adaptation

In coping with afflictions of the will, or just plain coherence of action, we move away from the possibility of endless choice—we limit both our perspective and our options. One mechanism by which we do this is the precommitments we make toward a course of action (Elster, 1979, 1999, 2000). These precommitments help bind us to the decisions we make and to the commitments that are the very heart of life in the world. "Taming chance" (Hacking, 1990), in part, reflects the choices that we make, the patterns of behavior that we establish, the part of our lives over which we have some control (Hacking, 1965, 1979; Peirce 1878/1992a, 1878/1992b, 1892/1992c).

As desires become overpowering, they compromise our practical inferences and habits, which is why the precommitments need to predominate and restrict choice. Rationality, as defined by Elster (2000; Fig. 6.3), must have means to satisfy these desires, and the beliefs themselves must be rational (Badgaiyan, 2000; Bargh et al., 2001; Wertenbroch, 1998).

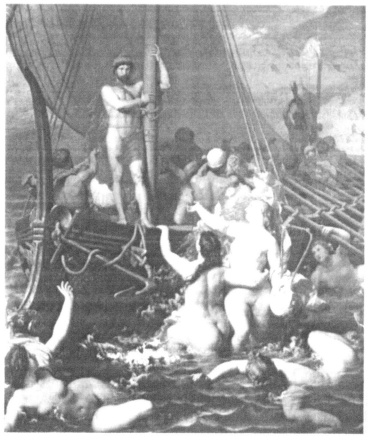

FIG. 6.3.   Ulysses.

One list of precommitments, as Elster (2000) has laid them out, includes the following:

1. Reducing options
2. Imposing costs
3. Establishing rewards
4. Creating timelines
5. Tagging preferences
6. Investing in bargaining
7. Reducing knowledge
8. Enhancing certain passions

Of course one should understand these commitments in the context, normally, of trying to balance risk taking amid a sane stable background; otherwise, one can be reduced to puritanical mediocrity.

Elster then provides an interesting analysis of strategies that might be effective in taking less in the short term and more in the long term in the rational adjudication of decision making for those vulnerable to alcohol consumption. They include the following:

1. Throwing away the key (no access)
2. Penalties
3. Creating diverse rewards
4. Creating delays
5. Changing beliefs
6. Avoiding exposure
7. Seeking good company

Making contracts and abiding by them is at the heart of our cultural ascent (Buchanan, 1975). Liberty is what many of us prize, but sanity emerges by the individual choice of living up to our promises, abiding by our contracts, and avoiding anarchy and the descent into the madness of choice.

Of course, for many individuals, all strategies can be tossed aside in seconds when the impulse to drink or consume a drug arises. But effective strategies are part of the armament of sane recovery, of pursuing wellness despite the pulls and pushes of salacious seduction. In the context of the vulnerable addict, the loss of flexibility of precommitments (Elster, 1979, 2000) by the limited range of rational action is obvious, as it should be for all of us. Abject freedom, the madness of choice (Sartre, 1948, 1956), must be combined with constraints of various sorts. In the context of ordinary life, getting through the imposition of chosen constraints is part of the rules of good conduct, of an effective will, if in the end it is to be effective and have meaning. This is age-old wisdom dressed in a modern vernacular. This is no trivial task, and there are better and worse methods for sustaining the course of action.

There are a variety of strategies that reflect our precommitments and a number of effective strategies that are self-binding and that protect us from poor choices and impulsive responses (Elster, 2000). Thus, to divert inconsistent action, to stay the course, Ulysses had himself bound to the mast of his ship. He needed to resist the Sirens' calls. The metaphors must be binding, the imagery large, and the force great to keep us on task.

As Elster has elegantly expressed, we precommit and take less in order to have more in some contexts, though certainly not all. Self-binding is just one strategy among others in overcoming our afflictions, in sustaining our intended goals, in organizing our lives toward rational self-regulation rather than bestial consumption. Ulysses tied to the mast is a metaphor for staying the course, staying sane in the face of that which can seduce us from our long-term goals. Some of us do not learn this lesson. As Cicero (1991) reminds us, "How many things Ulysses suffered during his lengthy wanderings" (p. 44). He was vulnerable to the seduction of the opposite sex. Metaphors play a wide range of cognitive functions (e.g., Lakoff, 1987) and in this context reflect the importance of self-binding commitments for our sanity (Siegel & Rachlin, 1996).

We seek to bind, sometimes by the invention of constitutional rules, to keep us committed to events that we know we should be committed to and working toward. This is one of the ways in which we fight our afflictions and addictions. It is an effective component of our mental hardware for ensuring that we do what we want to do, or at least what is better for us to do. Of course, the utter failure to fulfill these obligations is an everyday occurrence (Ariely & Wertenbroch, 2002; Becker & Murphy, 1988; Schelling, 2002).

Addictions and other afflictions compromise the will. Of course, many variants of good old-fashioned weakness of will can be discerned in both contemporary and classical literature (e.g., Davidson, 1969). Sometimes, apparent weakness gets lumped with poor reasoning and with deficient motivated systems. Within the context to which Elster points lies an omnipresent feature of our lives—namely, "addiction arises as the result of voluntary choices; once established, it undermines the capacity to choose or at least make rational choices" (Elster, 1999, p. 190).

DETECTION OF DISCREPANCY AND THE PREDICTION OF REWARD

Probability reasoning places the mind and the body back into adaptation. Probability reasoning reflects, perhaps, a specific mechanism in the cognitive arsenal for understanding the world that one is trying to cope with and understand. It is a mechanism that evolved to detect danger, to detect discrepancies, and then to generate new forms of committed behaviors. We might legitimately ask how and to what extent mechanisms were designed to predict predators and prey, food sources, and sexual success. With probability reasoning, prediction for one set of circumstances extended to new domains in our evolutionary ascent as our cognitive apparatus extended and expanded.

When expectations are thwarted, a broad array of learning occurs through new problem-solving search principles. This idea is close in scope to Peirce's (1878/1992a) view of inquiry and the development of new solutions to problems. Of course, inquiry is more than a mechanism for problem solving. In the 1970s, an important set of learning equations was developed which stated that not all learning is coupled to contingencies, and time of occurrence is not an axiomatic factor in learning, per se, but rather for predicting events (Rescorla, 1988; Rescorla & Wagner, 1972). This view of inquiry and learning was prescient, for the variants of this view would capture learning theory through what became known as the Rescorla–Wagner equation:

$$\Delta V = \alpha \beta (\lambda - V)$$

The Rescorla–Wagner model depicts the associative strengths of stimuli and how discrepancies from expectations are resolved. An association, and thereby learning, occurs by the strength of the predictions that are being developed. The model, then, not only becomes a mathematical approach to neural science but also incorporates a cognitive point of view. In the equation, V represents the current associative strength of the stimulus, while λ shows the maximum associative strength of the primary motivating event. The salience of conditioned and unconditioned stimuli are represented by α and β, respectively. The predictability of the primary motivating event is shown in the $(\lambda - V)$ term. When the current and maximum associative strengths of the stimulus are equal, the conditioned stimulus fully predicts the reinforcer. However, when the term is positive (λ is greater than V), the associative strength increases and the conditioned stimulus does not fully predict the reinforcer—and there is room for learning to occur. With increased associative strength, learning will occur and, in fact, occurs only ($\lambda - V$) term occurs when there is a loss of associative strength, and the predicted reinforcer fails (extinction).

This model is linked to events in learning in which prediction decreases learning (Rescorla & Wagner, 1972). Of course, large contexts of learning (incidental) do not entail this form of learning, which takes place by disruption of expectation. Disruption or discrepancy is a broad behavioral category (Kagan, 2002). The transmitter dopamine is involved in the organization or mobilization of behavioral responses. Again, effort is required, a sense of carrying through our actions, which is a good marker of the will.

DOPAMINE, DISCREPANCY, STRIATUM, AMYGDALA, AND THE FRONTAL CORTEX

As I have indicated previously, dopamine is an important neurotransmitter involved in both action and thought and, as such, is a necessary chemical information molecule in maintaining a coherent world in which to function (Kelley, 1999, 2004). Dopamine, for some time, has been linked to various features of reward (Wise, 2002, 2005).

Dopamine is not simply a neurotransmitter underlying the brain mechanisms linked to reward. It is much more complex. Even when dopamine is blocked, animals can still like things (e.g., sucrose; Berridge, 2004). Dopamine expression is essential for incentive motivation—the range of associations that is generated in terms of objects to approach or avoid (Berridge & Robinson, 1998; Spanagel & Weiss, 1999). The induction of dopamine in regions of the brain underlies the organization of action and increases the propensity to perform a number of psychological functions.

Central dopamine activation can occur when expectations are thwarted. In experiments in macaques, in which neurons were recorded electrophysiologically (Schultz, 2002; Schultz, Dayan, & Montague, 1997; Fig. 6.4), dopamine acti-

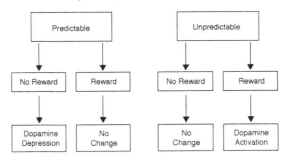

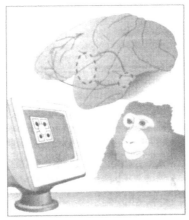

FIG. 6.4.   Reward and dopamine expression. (Top) Reprinted from *Neuron*, *36*, W. Schultz, Getting formal with dopamine and reward, 241–263, copyright © 2002, with permission from Elsevier. (Bottom) Reprinted from *Science*, *299*, P. Shizgal & A. Arvanitogiannis, Gambling on dopamine, 301, copyright © 2003, with permission from AAAS.

vation decreased with the repeated acquisition of an object and increased when an expectation was thwarted. Sets of dopaminergic neurons are activated in response to the perceived probability of a reward and are tied to the learning of these relationships. With a greater degree of likelihood, there is less dopamine activation. This places expectations and prediction of reward in a pivotal position, which brings reward, learning, and motivation in line with one another, though they are not axiomatically related.

But there are other sets of dopamine neurons that are less phasic and more tonic in their responses. Again, in macaques, activity in this second set of neurons is increased as the reward is anticipated. There is an increased activation toward the onset of the reward. Perhaps this set of neurons is more closely coupled with the motivational pull of the reward (Florillo et al., 2003). As Florillo et al. (2003) nicely put it, "The goal of learning can be seen as finding accurate predictors for motivationally significant events" (p. 1901). While other neurotransmitters are involved in the organization of learning and action, it is interesting that dopamine, so essential in the organization of movement, is also essential in the organization of thought and, in this case, the prediction of events (Fig. 6.5).

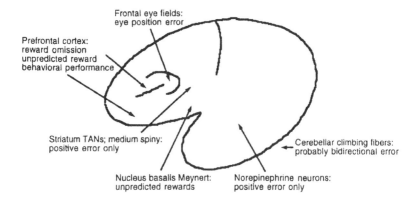

FIG. 6.5.   Neural structures responsive to error and uncertainty. Reprinted from *Neuron, 36,* W. Schultz, Getting formal with dopamine and reward, 241–263, copyright © 2002 with permission from Elsevier.

Dopamine neurons are linked to learning in a number of paradigms and in response to novel events (Tremblay, Hollerman, & Schultz, 1998) and knotted to the predicted value of the reward (Tobler, Florillo, & Schultz, 2005). Dopamine is important for focused attention and for facilitating memory processing (Roozendaal et al., 2001). In both animal and human studies, low doses of a dopamine agonist facilitate memory. Several regions of the brain are involved in this phenomenon, including the striatum and basal lateral amygdala (Roozendaal et al., 2001). The activation of central dopamine facilitates the learning of associations and the incentives, or range of associations (Berridge & Robinson, 1998), that figure in memory and the prediction of reward. The nucleus accumbens, for example, is linked to both positive and negative predictive choices (Roitman et al., 2005; Wakabayashi, Fields, & Nicola, 2004). Thus, when presented with reward events, dopamine neurons in the frontal cortex and striatum are active in anticipation and prediction of reward. Before a reward is fully predictable (i.e., the animal knows to expect it), one set of dopamine neurons are activated each time the reward is given. And thus, for this set of dopamine neurons, once the reward is predictable (i.e., always occurring without failure), dopamine no longer is activated (Schultz et al., 1997). In other words, as the event becomes less novel, so too does the firing of these neurons.

Other interpretations of the anticipatory dopamine response have tied it to attentional resources and to motivational events (Horvitz, 2000). And decision making often involves attributing value to events that predict rewards. Two regions of the brain are involved: the frontal cortex and striatum (Montague & Berns, 2002). Brain imaging studies reveal activation of these regions when decisions about rewards are being made (O'Doherty et al., 2001) and when rewards are being predicted (Breiter et al., 2001).

In one study, positron emission tomography (PET) was used to measure brain activity in human subjects in a "go/no-go" task. Correct responses were reinforced with the possibility of a monetary reward in one group, whereas another group was simply asked to say "okay." The possibility of reward was associated with greater activation in the dorsal prefrontal cortex (Thut et al., 1997). The expectation of the reward mattered. Other investigators studying expectations of monetary losses and gains consistently find activation in these same areas of the cortex, in addition to the striatum, amygdala, and other regions of the brain (e.g., Breiter et al., 2001).

Moreover, regions of the orbitofrontal and cingulate cortex, the paradigmatic structures that underlie a broad array of human reasoning and problem solving, are grounded by visceral input that informs judgment. Damage to these regions impairs anticipatory responses in a variety of contexts (Bechara et al., 2002; Damasio, 1994, 1999). For example, in experiments in which control subjects and patients with frontal lobe damage were compared in a gambling test, the sensitivity to risk—the autonomic representation of risk—was correlated with correct decision making in a variety of experimental contexts (Bechara, 2005). Control subjects who generated risky strategies on these gambling tasks in the choice between advantageous and disadvantageous card decks revealed greater anticipatory skin conductance than did the patients with frontal lobe damage. The important observation from this study is that changes in skin conductance, measures of autonomic, peripheral input, are apparent before decision making occurs in normal subjects on a number of these experimental paradigms, but such changes are not seen in those subjects in which the visceral cortical representations have been damaged or destroyed and their judgment diminished or compromised (Bechara, 2005; Damasio, 1994).

Other studies have provided a wide variety of examples that demonstrate relationships between reasoning about probability and the activation of a wide network of structures in the brain, including diverse cortical and subcortical sites (Knowlton et al., 1996; Thut et al., 1997). These studies have shown that representations of future monetary rewards activate regions of the orbitofrontal cortex (O'Doherty et al., 2001).

CONCLUSION

Effort and the will are essential to decision making (e.g., long-term gains from short-term satisfaction). One behavioral strategy is to organize our willed actions according to the commitments or precommitments that we make: the precommitments to rise in the morning to swim, to run, to write, and so forth. Expectations of reward figure in the organization of the will and in the cognitive assessment that underlies the organization of action. Predicting future events, including rewards, is part of the cognitive machinery embodied in regions of the brain such as the frontal cortex and basal ganglia.

When choice is demythologized (from the pedestal of perfect reason) good-enough problem solving is the only available option. One important behavioral strategy is to bind ourselves to a set of behaviors oriented to our goals and to group our decisions that increase our willpower. It is a strategy bound to create behavioral coherence (e.g., Ainslie, 2001; Elster, 1979, 2000), but of course it has to be linked to the right sorts of ends (Dewey, 1925/1989; Neville, 1974).

We, and other species, are probability generators. This capacity allows us to organize our behavior so as to predict reward, to focus attention, and to achieve goals. The prediction of reward, expectancies that underlie behavioral expression, requires dopamine regulation in the central nervous system. This cognitive ability, and the greater control over our behavioral options that it affords, is importantly linked to our sense of effort and the will, sustaining a chosen direction amid endless conflict.

Conclusion: An Understanding of Effort and the Will

Several propositions inhere in our thinking about effort and the will in the context of the brain: our capacity to choose and to limit choice and stay bound to a course, our will reflects the evolution of our brain and our biology (Dretske, 1994; Flanagan, 1984; Goldman, 1970; Glynn, 1999). We are creatures with a complex biology but with some room to move; we have exorbitant amounts of creative flair, and also the potential for destructive force.

Just as William James noted that consciousness is not a thing, memory is not a thing (Eichenbaum & Cohen, 2001). The will is also not a thing. The will serves many functions (Pink, 1996) and is essential in diverse adaptive capacities, including basic regulatory motivations that are essential for bodily regulation, the ontogeny of behavioral inhibition, and the adjudication of long- and short-term goals. Thus, effort or the will is a product of many neural systems designed to operate and cooperate in the organization of behavior. There is no one system designed for the will. Nor does it make much sense to talk about multiple wills. That would bring on the absurd and be more than enough reason to throw out the concept. However, there are different subcomponents of what we take the will to be built from, some of which I have sketched in each chapter.

The will functions in our lexicon of legitimacy like a number of other important traditional concepts (e.g., intention), namely, to explain and predict behavior. My relying on your capacity to carry out what you say you will do requires me to attribute something like a will to you, particularly when it requires effort. There is nothing make-believe or mythical about this. It is fundamental to us (Kane, 2002).

The expression of the will is perhaps partly found in the innervation of dopaminergic function and the onset of behavioral inhibition and behavioral control (Diamond, 2001; Young, Joseph, & Gray, 1993). The will allows us to make the link between decision making and needs and to postpone certain present needs for the future satisfaction that fits one's longer term interests—to learn to delay gratification (Mischel & Mischel, 1987; Mischel, Shoda, & Rodriguez, 1989). The breakdown of the will is reflected in the pathologies that emerge: obsessive-compulsive disorder, schizophrenia, and a wide variety of afflictions that reflect diseases and dissolution of the nervous system. They reflect a family of factors in which one can see the dissolution of the will. In this conclusion to the book, I reiterate some earlier themes about neuroscience, that is, the sense of effort and self-control and the idea that the exercise of the will, like other behavioral and physiological functions, is subject to fatigue (Baumeister & Vohs, 2003; Binswanger, 1992; Brandstatter et al., 2001)

A NEUROSCIENTIFIC PERSPECTIVE

Behavioral neuroscience is still in its infancy. Though its rudiments can be traced back thousands of years, it has propelled us forward only in the past two centuries, and in particular the past 40 years. Intellectually relocating the organ of the mind from the periphery (heart) to the brain was one of the first advances. From there we began to explore the functioning of the brain in terms of our wants, desires, and thoughts, and our capacity to control them. This major advance (Hippocrates) was accompanied by the idea that neuroscientific investigation should focus on the nerves and the structure of the brain (Galen, Vesalius, see Bota et al., 2003; Finger, 1994; Gross, 1999; Swanson, 2003) and dividing the motor regions of the brain into voluntary and involuntary functions (Finger 1994; Swanson, 2003).

Although interest in the nervous system is ancient (Gross, 1999), it is only within the last 150 years that our structural and chemical understanding of the nervous system has developed (Kandel & Squire, 2000). From seeing neurons to understanding the mechanisms of the synapse, we know something about the cellular organization of the brain. Perhaps the most profound work has been that of linking biology to cognition—from cell to computational design.

One place in which these events have taken place is in the understanding of the cellular mechanisms—the role of dopamine in various aspects of movement and cognition. Dopaminergic function has long been known and has been studied in a number of systems over the last 30 years (e.g., Mogenson & Huang, 1973; Montague et al., 1996); central dopamine expression underlies basic control functions that underlie attentional mechanisms that are essential in the organization of action (Norman & Shallice, 1980), motivation and outcomes (Satoh et al., 2003) in which the detection of unexpected salience (Dommett et al., 2005) or simply incentive salience (Berridge & Robinson, 1998), novelty (Horvitz, 2000), uncertainty and learning (Niv, Duff, & Dayan, 2005), anticipation (Suri, 2001) and the prediction of events and the context figure importantly (cf., Nakahara et al., 2004; Redgrave, Prescott, & Gurney, 1999; Schultz, 2002). Both prefrontal cortex and regions of the basal ganglia are involved in the organization of behavior that underlies reward-related behaviors (e.g., Zald et al., 2004). Central dopamine probably underlies most aspects of the organization of behavior, including reproductive behaviors (Champagne et al., 2004). Dopamine levels in the nucleus accumbens contribute toward partner preference (Aragona et al., 2003) and altering the genes that regulate dopamine expression results in behavioral changes that underlie partner preference (Lim et al., 2004). Underlying the attentional, the associative, and the predictive mechanisms are sustaining instrumental behaviors, in which dopamine regulation is essential. Central dopamine expression is neutral with regard to positive or aversive stimuli and is involved in both kinds of events (Pruessner et al., 2004; Ungless, Magill, & Botam, 2004) and in the prediction of reward (Schultz, 2002; Wakabayashi et al., 2004). An important point that figures throughout the book is that central dopamine underlies diverse forms of behavioral regulation—both appetitive and aversive events result in the central expression of dopamine.

Any neuroscience perspective needs to take into account the origins of the development of the nervous system (e.g., Changeux & Cahavaillon, 1995). Corticalization of function is just one feature of our evolutionary ascent; another is the increased access to the brain stem and the greater use of specialized preadaptive mechanisms (Holloway, 1995; Mayr, 1982; Rozin, 1998). The greater innervation of the brain stem and direct access of the cortex to the brain stem increase the range of behavioral and physiological options available to us.

The brain is prepared to express diverse forms of motor behavior, which are permeated with cognitive expectations (e.g., Dewey, 1896; Jeannerod, 1988; Lotze, 1852; Prinz, 2003). Increased access to the lower brain stem increases our self-control and self-discipline—key features in holding present desires at bay and being able to regulate and keep intact our long-term desires (Schulkin, 2003; Sterling, 2004).

It is now commonplace to depict decision making in both animal and human neuroscientific literature. Part of this change reflects the rise of the cognitive sciences and the recognition that competing cognitive resources are utilized in problem-solving situations. Underlying the utilization of information-processing systems is the neurotransmitter dopamine, which figures in all aspects of cognition, including motor control and behavior.

A PERSPECTIVE ON EFFORT AND THE WILL

Evolution has provided enough "elbow room" (Dennett, 1999, 2003) for an evolving human freedom, a crowning achievement of our species, culminating in cultures that allow us to attain responsibility (Kane, 1998, 2002) and have diverse choices (Neville, 1974). As Dennett (2003) rightly notes, "Free will is real" (p. 13), but it is not given; it is an achievement, a combination of cephalic and social/ecological co-evolution.

The problem that I set out to solve was to give the will a more naturalized sense by (a) suggesting that cognitive systems are inherent in the organization of action, the expression of the will reflecting information processing or cognitive systems in the central nervous system; and (b) suggesting that central dopamine and traditional motor areas are importantly tied to cognitive systems in the organization of action. I have emphasized central dopamine because it is a candidate for this functional role; dopamine is only one information molecule among others in the organization of behavior (Herbert & Schulkin, 2002).

The conception of the will as "the varieties worth having," to borrow from Dennett (1999, 2003), shows its face in diverse ways. Underlying many of the considerations of the will is that we hold each other accountable. The solution of reducing the issue of the will to the way in which we use language (Anscombe, 1957; Austin, 1961; Ryle, 1949) is a useful exercise in clarifying what is at stake and in avoiding confusion. But unless one still holds that it is simply a question of language use, namely, considerations of the will, and that there is no real fact of the matter, then the inquiry stops there.

I personally find the Stoic conception of the will to be the most congenial, laced with modern notions of self-determination, coupled with a sense of evolving, surviving individuals trying to cope and make sense of their surroundings. The endless plight for us is being thrown into a particular context by birth and circumstance and then making sense of it: coping, living, and even trying to thrive.

There is nothing ghostly about considerations of the will in the above-lived context, no bogeyman. There are pockets of indeterminacy, in which giving a value to the variable under discussion is difficult, sometimes impossible, to determine. The concept figures in the practices that permeate our everyday transactions. The drive for self-expression and for regulatory control evolved together in our cultural development. But this does not mean that there are little people in our heads or that we have special access to most of the cognitive processing with regard to conscious control. There are, however, specific and less specific problem-solving programs in our brains designed to carve out coherence. The elements of sustained activation and control, inhibition, and coordinated adaptive responses are to be found in this self-regulation and self-control.

We want to capture the myriad ways in which we express ourselves, persist in our actions, and take responsibility for our choices and our actions. We want to demythologize the drama of choice. Practical abilities are tied to our choices, as is practical reason and knowing how to do things and how to avoid things. The development of reason is linked to the practices of life, and the ability to do things is tied to the will, to our choices, and to our responsibility for what we are (Stroud & Tappolet, 2003).

The issue for the consideration of the will is that one could have done differently, that it was not ordained and that choice was an option (Frankfurt, 1988). To deny choice and free will is to throw out our show. We need to demythologize the drama of absolute freedom versus brute determinism and scale it down to human proportions. Choice is expressed under conditions of diverse constraints, in which diverse conflicting desires and interests compete for expression, in which the cognitive resources are caught in tangled webs that can and do impede coherent action.

As Dennett (1984, 1999) nicely puts it, "The varieties of free will we deem worth wanting are those—if there are any—that will secure for us our dignity and responsibility" (p. 152). This is where demythologized reason, not lofty abstract and divorced reason, needs its soulmate, a demythologized concept of the will. No mystification is necessary with the adequate and appropriate use of the concept.

One common discussion of the will turns to setting and sustaining commitments, and bargaining and then sustaining longer term goals. The will takes its shape, as James (1899/1958) understood, "full of scruples and inhibitions" (p. 122). James was always searching for the positive message. But excessive inhibition and repressive control are the drama of the self trying to master itself, overcoming vulnerability to anxiety, hysteria, and obsessive-compulsive addictions (Freud, 1926/1959). Part of the self-fulfillment of understanding is moving beyond and struggling throughout with the drama of what is under control, what is subject to our will (Augustine, 1964; Aurelius, 1964; Camus, 1955; Freud, 1895; Hume, 1739/1964; Sabini & Silver, 1986; Seneca, 1969; Sidgwick, 1907/1981).

Any real sense of volition has to include something of the individual knowing something about what she wants, what she is striving for (Kenny, 1998), but that is not to say that all aspects of the will are conscious. In fact, most pervasive and cephalic operations are outside of our awareness. The great cognitive arsenal is mostly unconscious (Rozin, 1998); the same goes for what we call the "conscious will" (Wegner, 2002). Many sorts of illusions surround our experience of the will (Wegner, 2002). But then there are many sorts of illusions that surround our perceptual systems. We are not likely to discard the concept of perception. Similarly, our notion of the will is not something to be given up, like belief in witches. Illusions are one thing; giving up on the concept is quite another. We have learned that we are quite limited in our introspective determination of what makes us do what we do, and the will is no different in that regard from many other mental events. We are not simply looking in on some causal machinery that we have normally called the will. If we take this route, then surely the end result is disappointing.

There is little doubt that the concept of the will, despite the protestations of the most scientific of us, is fundamental to our folk conception of ourselves in addition to its link in the science of brain function and behavioral organization. I have not tried to solve the dilemma of determinism versus freedom (see Kane, 1998, for the many variants of arguments as they pertain to our notion of the will). And it is important to note the diverse ways in which we can be misled about our understanding of our actions, the causation of behaviors and the illusions and mistaken ideas that we have—and this goes for making events occur through the power of the will (Wegner, 2002). Wegner is right that mechanisms generating our sense of having a will are not the same as our experience of willing.

I have chosen to capture what is intelligible about the concept and to draw some of the neuroscientific and behavioral literature in line with our considerations of the will. This is no easy fit, and others no doubt will do a better job of it. The commonsense cluster of factors associated with the will is something worth preserving as we proceed ahead. But there is no simple map of how to link our commonsense notion of the will, naturalized within a psychobiological perspective, and the organization of the brain and its cognitive machinations. The issue is less about what is transparent to the individual and more about the way in which we explain the organization of action and the cognitive, neural, and ecological mechanisms that make this possible.

My strategy has been to demythologize our notion of the will, rendering it less ethereal, less vulnerable to elimination from our scientific tendencies, mine included. We want to understand the conceptual space for our folk psychological depiction. Our range of choices has accrued with our evolutionary ascent and the cultural context in which we find and make ourselves, as has our freedom (Dennett, 2003; Dewey, 1925/ 1989).

We live with conflicted appetites, values, and desires. Movement, as Aristotle long noted in animals, is driven by both appetites and reason; the distinction is not as great as he thought. Cognitive systems permeate the appetites, the valuation of events. Cognition is not one side and willing on the other.

Of course, dissolving the issue, not from a conceptual legitimacy of the everyday but from a scientific blade of expediency and parsimony, certainly has its merits (Churchland, 2002). The endless confusion surrounding the concept of will and its indeterminacy and inaccuracies in use raises the fury of any scientific sensibility. But this is shortsighted, unless we have something with which to replace the concept of will. I don't think we have that yet.

I suppose one could, as some do, or not hold onto the view that free will is an essential illusion—that we are forced to hold the concept while acknowledging the nonreality of the will (cf., Double, 1991; Honderich, 2002; Smilansky, 2000). Living with an illusion is a prelude to rationality in decision making, holding people accountable. I prefer acknowledging the reality of the will (see also Dupre, 1996; Libet, 1985, 2004).

AN IMPORTANT PIECE OF US: WILLING

Voluntary action, motivation, and self-control are core features of human freedom and human decision making (e.g., Jaspers, 1913/1997). In one form or another, as argued by many thinkers, our core feature is that of holding ourselves responsible (Kane, 1998). Issues within the psychology of human decision making are the expression of effort (James, 1890/1952) and self-control and the practical iterations with the world we are trying to understand and adapt to. The power of efficacy of choice rests on some sense of the will (Kane, 1998). Naturalizing the will is placing this efficacy in an evolutionary context, one of greater control over behavior, a greater range of options, and so on.

But fortune matters—the pervasive chance meetings, chance events. There is the gambling aspect of everyday life, the wheel out of our control (Fig. C.1). In staying the course, disciplined will is essential in the face of a wheel that is often out of our control.

Naturalizing the will can be elucidated through examples of dissolution of the nervous system's competency—its breakdown in a number of disease states of the brain (e.g., schizophrenia). The will is rooted in our understanding of the information-processing systems in the brain. The language of the brain is limited and does not capture the richness of the concept, but considerations of the will in the end must and should refer back to the functioning of the brain, under both normal and pathological conditions.

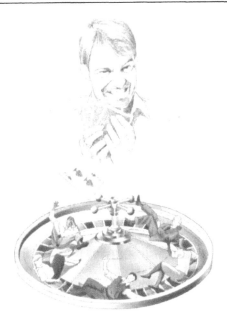

FIG. C.1.   Gambler.

The will, when posed in good faith as a philosophical problem, is perhaps not solvable (McGinn, 1997, 1999), and this
has forced us to think clearly about whether we solve philosophical dilemmas (e.g., the problem of consciousness). So
too is the consideration of the will perhaps a reminder that,
although there are no ghosts in the machinery, the machinery
is not all that we are trying to understand. That having been
said, there is an epistemological humility that should be in-
voked: The concept of the will is a troublesome one.

Several issues dominate the discussion of the will. Did we
choose to act in a way we wanted? Does the choice make sense
relative to the background and context? Could we have done
otherwise (Frankfurt, 1971)? And, did the choice have some
primary locus in the individual (Walter, 2001)? Whether historical or biological, the conception of inevitability for a wide
range of human actions has been demythologized and sized
down to a human proportion replete with choice and
circumstance and Fortuna.

The will, as a number of investigators have noted, is not simply noticed before an action. But neither is the will something I discover about myself only after the act (e.g., Prinz, 2003). On this view, by necessity, I don't discover that I am willing something until I notice the effort. It is, perhaps, something like the mistaken Jamesian notion of finding out that I am afraid because I am running. I can be afraid and run or not run. I can imagine instances in which I might not know that I am willing something, so distracted by events that I am not aware of what I am doing. But of course that need not be, and often is not, the case. Despite the fact that many still might believe that introspection says something about the will (e.g., Nathan, 1992), I think, as Prinz (2003) has suggested, that there may be no special privileged epistemological sense of my understanding my will from my understanding yours; I, or you, can be equally wrong judging our selves, or judging one other.

One feature of our evolution, as I have indicated, is the expression of cognitive fluidity or flexibility (Mitchen, 1996), along with a conception of the will in cultural terms shorn of its mythological glorification and now knotted to our understanding of the organization of action and our evolution. Many diverse thinkers have suggested that cognitive systems are endemic to motor systems (e.g., Holst, 1973; Hommel, 1996). Diverse studies suggest that action words, for example, activate regions of the motor cortex (e.g., Hauk et al., 2004; Pulvermuller, Shtyrov, & Ilmoniemi, 2005), that cognitive systems are found throughout diverse systems in the brain. Moreover, we know that cognitive systems can be reflexive and triggered.

One very important feature of the will is the inhibition of behavior, in which there is no action except the inhibition of doing something (e.g., not smoking). The will is integral to the realization of our goals and plans. Our understanding of human agency and human action is rich in the use of the concept of the will (Neville, 1974). That does not mean that the will or other concepts, such as motivation, are identical to specific regions of the brain. Endemic to our concept of human action is the linking of desires and beliefs with abilities and opportunities (Goldman, 1970, 1990). One mechanism is the precommitment that binds, that facilitates control (Elster, 1999, 2000) and anchors one to the cognitive resources embedded in our social environment (Clark, 1999), and that creates categories of decisions that provide for coherent action that reflects one's long-term goals (Ainslie, 2001, 2005).

There is no split between regions of the brain that are cognitive and those that are motor. There are, however, different kinds of cognitive systems, some of which are knotted to motor systems, and those that are not, some are conscious, most are not, some reach the cortex, others do not. This allows one, perhaps, to understand how the will functions in our lexicon for systems that facilitate the adaptive nature of behavioral options, the choices that we make.

From the point of view of our experience, these are the moments of coming into being (Whitehead, 1927; see also Dennett, 2003; Neville, 1974), of sustaining oneself in the face of the goals to be pursued. Our evolution reflects the greater range of choices, the greater ability to self-bind against those events worthy of avoiding or stay the course for future behaviors. James highlighted the sense of effort in the everyday sense of life and also a will that matters in the face of the interests of other people and other external objects. This was poetically noted by diverse thinkers from Wordsworth to Whitehead—the sense of willing into being is perhaps followed by a sense of decay or entropy with the breakdown of systems not made to last: What remains is a stoic sense that the act itself is worthy when directed to goals that enhance the human condition. But amid the great triumphs of human expression are the diverse ways in which we have trampled on one other, sustained the wrong goals, and directed the will toward the less worthy at the expense of others.

REFERENCES

Adey, W. R. (1974). Information processing and I sensory and motor systems. In W. R. Adey et al., (Eds.), *Brain mechanisms and the control of behaviour* (pp. 326–342). London: Heinemann.

Ainslie, G. (1975). Specious reward: A behavioral theory of impulsiveness and impulse control. *Psychological Bulletin, 82,* 463–496.

Ainslie, G. (1999). The dangers of willpower: A picoeconomic understanding of addiction and dissociation. In J. Elster & O.-J. Skog (Eds.), *Getting hooked: Rationality and addiction* (pp. 65–92). Cambridge, UK: Cambridge University Press.

Ainslie, G. (2001). *Breakdown of will.* Cambridge, UK: Cambridge University Press.

Ainslie, G. (2005). Precis of breakdown of will. *Behavioral & Brain Sciences, 28,* 635–673.

Ainslie, G., & Monterosso, J. (2003). Hyperbolic discounting as a factor in addiction: A critical review. In N. Heather & R. E. Vuchinich (Eds.), Choice, behavioural economics, and addiction (pp. 35–62).

Ainslie, G., & Monterosso, J. (2004). A marketplace in the brain? *Science, 306,* 421–423.

Aldridge, J. W., & Berridge, K. C. (1998). Coding of serial order by neostriatal neurons: A natural action approach to move sequence. *Journal of Neuroscience, 18*, 2777–2787.

Aldridge, J. W. & Berridge, K. C. (2002). Coding of behavioral sequences in the basal ganglia. In L. F. B. Nicolson & R. L. Faull (Eds.), *The basal ganglia* (Vol. 7, pp 53–66). New York: Kluwer Academic/Plenum.

Aldridge, J. W., Berridge, K. C., Herman, M., & Zimmer, L. (1993). Neuronal coding of serial order: Syntax of grooming in the neostratum. *Psychological Science, 4*, 391–393.

Alexander, G. E., Crutcher, M. D., & DeLong, M. R. (1991). Basal ganglia thalamocortical circuits: Parallel substrates for motor, oculomotor, prefrontal, and limbic functions. *Progress in Brain Research, 85*, 119–145.

Alheid, G. F., & Heimer, L. (1988). New perspectives in basal forebrain organization of special relevance for neuropsychiatric disorders: The striatopallidal, amygdaloid, and corticopetal components of substantia innominata. *Neuroscience, 27*, 1–39.

Andreasen, N.C., Arndt, S., Alliger, R., Mller, D., & Flaum, M. (1999). Symptoms of schizophrenia: Methods, meanings, and mechanisms. *Archives of General Psychiatry, 52*, 341–351.

Anscombe, G. E. M. (1957). *Intention*. Oxford, UK: Blackwell.

Aragona, B. J., Yan-Liu, J., Curtis, T., Stephan, F. K., & Wang, Z. (2003). A critical role for nucleus accumbens dopamine in partner-preference formation in male prairie voles. *Journal of Neuroscience, 23*, 3483–3490.

Arbib, M. A. (1981). Perceptual structures and distributed motor control. In V. B. Brooks (Ed.), *Handbook of Physiology*, Section 2: The nervous system, Vol. 2: Motor control (Pt. 1, pp. 1449–1180). Baltimore: Williams & Wilkins.

Ariely, D., & Werrtenbroch, K. (2002). Procrastination, deadlines, and performance: self-control by precommitment. *Psychological Science, 13*, 219–224.

Aristotle. (1974). *Ethics*. New York: Penguin Books.

Augustine. (1964). *On the free choice of the will*. Indianapolis: Bobbs-Merrill.

Aurelius, Marcus (1964). *Meditations*. London, UK: Penguin Books.

Austin, J. L. (1961). Ifs and cans. In J. O. Urmson & G. Warnock (Eds.), *Philosophical papers* (pp.153–180). Oxford, UK: Clarendon Press.

Badgaiyan, R. D. (2000). Executive control, willed actions, and nonconscious processing. *Human Brain Mapping, 9*, 38–41.

Badre, D., & Wagner, A. D. (2004). Selection, integration and conflict monitoring: Assessing the nature and generality of prefrontal cognitive control mechanisms. *Neuron, 41*, 473–487.

Baimoukhametova, D. V., Hewitt, S. A., Sank, C. A., Bains, J. S. (2004). Dopamine modulates use-dependent plasticity of inhibitory synapses. *Journal of Neuroscience, 24,* 5162–5175.

Bain, A. (1859/1886). *The emotions and the will.* New York: Appleton.

Baker, C. A., & Morrison, A. P. (1998). Cognitive processes in auditory hallucinations. Attributional biases and metacognition. *Psychological Medicine, 28,* 1199–1208.

Bargh, J. A., Gollwitzer, P. M., Lee-Chai, A., Barndollar, K., & Trtschel, R. (2001). The automated will: nonconscious activation and pursuit of behavioral goals. *Journal of Personality and Social Psychology, 81,* 1014–1027.

Barlow, J. H., Cosmides, L., & Tooby, J. (1992). *The adapted mind.* Oxford, UK: Oxford University Press.

Baron, J. (2003). *Thinking and deciding* (3rd ed.). Cambridge, UK: Cambridge University Press.

Baron-Cohen, S. (1995). *Mindblindness.* Cambridge: MIT Press.

Baron-Cohen, S., Flusberg-Tager, H., & Cohen, D. J. (2000) *Understanding other minds* (2nd ed.). Oxford, UK: Oxford University Press.

Barr, L. C., Goodman, W. K., Price, L. H., McDougle, C. J., & Charney, D. S. (1992). The serotonin hypothesis of obsessive compulsive disorder: Implications of pharmacologic challenge studies. *Journal of Clinical Psychiatry, 54*(4), 17–28.

Baumeister, R. Y., & Vohs, K. D. (2003). Willpower, choice and self-control. In G. Loewenstein & D. Read (Eds.), *Time and decision: Economic and psychological perspectives on intertemporal choice* (pp. 42–62). New York: Sage Press.

Baxter, L. R., Jr. (2003). Basal ganglia systems in ritualistic social displays: reptiles and humans: function and illness. *Physiology and Behavior, 79,* 431–460.

Baxter, L. R., Jr., & Brody, A. (1996). Neuroimaging in obsessive-compulsive disorder: advances in understanding neuroanatomy, In H. G. M. Westenberg, J. A. Den Boer, & D. L. Murphy (Eds.), *Advances in the neurobiology of anxiety disorders* (pp. 329–348). New York: Wiley.

Bechara, A. (2005). Decision-making, impulse control and loss of willpower to resist drugs: A neurocognitive perspective. *Nature Neuroscience, 8,* 1458–1463.

Bechara, A., Dolan, S., & Hindes, A. (2002). Decision-making and addiction (Pt. II): Myopia for the future or hypersensitivity for reward? *Neuropsychologia, 40,* 1690–1705.

Bechara, A., Nader, K., van der Kooy, D. (1998). A two separate-motivational systems hypothesis of opioid addiction. *Pharmacology, Biochemistry and Behavior, 59,* 1–17.

Becker, G. S., & Murphy, K. (1988). A theory of rational addiction. *Journal of Political Economy 96*, 75–700.

Becker, J. B., Rudick, C. N., & Jenkins, W. J. (2000). The role of dopamine in the nucleus accumbens and striatum during sexual behavior in the female rat. *The Journal of Neuroscience, 21*, 3236–3241.

Bentham, J. (1948). *An introduction to the principles of morals and legislation*. Introduction by L. J. Lafleur. New York: Hafner Press. (Original work published 1789)

Bergson, H. (2001). *Time and free will*. New York: Dover Press. (Original work published 1913)

Berlin, I. (1969). *Four essays on liberty*. Oxford, UK: Oxford University Press.

Berns, G. S., McClure, S. M., Pagnoni, G., & Montague, P. R. (2001). Predictability modulates human brain response to reward. *Journal of Neuroscience, 21*(8) 2793–2798.

Berridge, K. C. (2004). Motivation concepts in behavioral neuroscience. *Physiology and Behavior, 81*, 179–209.

Berridge, K. C., & Aldridge, J. W. (2000). Super-sterotypy II: Enhancement of a complex movement sequence by intraventricular dopamine D1 agonists. *Synapse, 37*, 205–215.

Berridge, K. C., Aldridge, J. W., Houchard, K. H., & Zhuang, X. (2005). Sequential super-sterotypy of an instinctive fixed action pattern in hyper-dopaminergic mutant mice: A model of obsessive compulsive disorder and Tourette's. *BMC Biology, 2*, 1–16.

Berridge, K. C., Flynn, F. W., Schulkin, J., & Grill, H. J. (1984). Sodium depletion enhances salt palatability in rats. *Behavioral Neuroscience, 98*, 652–660.

Berridge, K. C., & Robinson, T. E. (1998). What is the role of dopamine in reward: Hedonic impact, reward learning or incentive salience? *Brain Research Reviews, 18*, 309–369.

Berridge, K. C. & Whitshaw, I. Q. (1992). Cortex, striatum, and cerebellum: Control of serial order in a grooming sequence. *Experimental Brain Research, 90*, 275–290.

Berrios, G. E., & Gili, M. (1995). Will and its disorders: A conceptual history. *History of Psychiatry, 6* (21, Pt.1), 87–104.

Berthoz, A., (2002). *The brain's sense of movement*. Cambridge, MA: Harvard University Press.

Binswanger, H. (1992). Volition as cognitive self-regulation. *Organizational Behavior & Human Decision Processes, 50*(2), 154–178.

Bizzi, E., & Mussa-Ivaldi, F. A. (2000). Toward a neurobiology of coordinate transformations. Chapter 34 In: The New Cognitive Neurosciences. , 2nd edition, M. S. Gazzaniga, Editor-in-chief. Cambridge.:Bradford Book, MIT Press.

Bjorklund, A., Divac, I., & Lindvall, O. (1978). Regional distribution of catecholamines in monkey cerebral cortex, evidence for a dopaminergic innervation of the primate prefrontal cortex. *Neuroscience Letters, 7,* 115–119.

Bjorklund, A., & Lindvall, O. (1984). Dopamine-containing systems in the CNS. In A. Bjorklund & T. Hokfelt (Eds.), Handbook of chemical neuroanatomy, Classical transmitters in the CNS (Pt. 1, Vol. 2, pp. 55–122). Amsterdam: Elsevier.

Blakemore, S. J., Oakley, D. A., & Frith, C. D. (2003). Delusions of alien control in the normal brain. *Neuropsychologia, 41,* 1058–1067.

Block, N. (1978). Troubles with functionalism. In C. W. Savage (Ed.), *Perception and cognition: Issues in the foundations of psychology,* (pp. 60–84). Minneapolis: University of Minnesota.

Bota, M., Dong, H. W., & Swanson, L. W. (2003). From gene networks to brain networks. *Nature Neuroscience, 6,* 795–799.

Brandstatter, V., Lengfelder, A., & Gollwitzer, P. M. (2001). Implementation intentions and efficient action initiation. *Journal of Personality and Social Psychology, 81,* 946–960.

Braver, T. S., Barch, D. M., & Cohen, J. D. (1999). Cognition and control in schizophrenia: A computational model of dopamine and prefrontal function. *Biological Psychiatry, 46,* 312–328.

Breiter, H. C., Aharon, I, Kahneman, D., Dale, A., & Shizgal, P. (2001). Functional imaging of neural responses to expectancy and experience of monetary gains and losses. *Neuron, 30(2),* 619–639.

Breiter, H. C., Gollub, R. L., Weiskoff, R. M., Kennedy, D. N., Makris, N., Berke, J. D., Goodman, J. M., Kantor, H. L., Gastfriend, D. R., Riorden, J. P., Mathew, R. T., Rosen, B. R., & Hyman, S. E. (1997). Acute effects of cocaine on human brain activity and emotion. *Neuron, 19,* 591–611.

Broca, P. (1863). *Localization des fonctions cérébrales. Siege du langage articulé. Bulletins de la Societé d'Anthropologie, 4,* 200–203.

Brodal, A. (1981). *Neurological anatomy* (3rd ed.). New York: Oxford University Press.

Brodmann, K. (1909). *Vergleichende Lokalisationslehre der Grosshirnrinde in ithren Prinzipien dargestellt auf Grund des Zellenbaues.* Leipzig: Barth.

Brown, B. M., Crane, A. M., & Goldman, P. S. (1976). Catecholamines in neocortex of rhesus monkeys. Regional distribution and ontogenetic development. *Brain Research, 124,* 576–580.

Brown, P., & Marsden, C. D. (1998). What do the basal ganglia do? *The Lancet, 351,* 1801–1894.

Brown, R. M., Crane, A. M., & Goldman, P. S. (1979). Regional distribution of monoamines in the cerebral cortex and subcortical structures of the rhesus monkey: Concentrations and in vivo synthesis rates. *Brain Research, 168,* 133–150.

Brunner, R. L., Jordan, M. K., & Berry, H. K. (1983). Early-treated phenylketonuria: Neuropsychologic consequences. *Journal of Pediatrics, 102,* 831–835.

Buccino, G., Vogt, S., Ritzi, A., Fink, G. R., & Zilles, G., (2004). Neural circuits underlying imitation learning of hand actions: An event related fMRI study. *Neuron, 42,* 323–334.

Buchanan, J. M. (1975). *The limits of liberty: Between anarchy and leviathan.* Chicago: University of Chicago Press.

Caine, S. B., Heinrichs, S. C., Coffin, V. L., & Koob, G. F. (1995). Effects of the dopamine D-1 antagonist SCH 23390 microinjected into the accumbens, amygdala or striatum on cocaine self-administration in the rat. *Brain Research, 692,* 47–46.

Cajal, S. R. (1906). The structure and connexions of neurons. In *Nobel Lectures, Physiology or Medicine 1901–1921* (pp. 220–253). New York: Elsevier.

Calder, A. J., Lawrence, A. D., & Young, A. W. (2001). Neuropsychology of fear and loathing. *Nature Neuroscience, 2,* 352–362.

Camerer, C., Loewenstein, G., Prelec, D. (2005). Neuroeconomics: How neuroscience can inform economics. *Journal of Economic Literature, 43,* 9–64.

Camus, A. (1955). *The myth of Sisyphus.* New York: Random House.

Cannon, C. M., & Palmiter, R. D. (2003). Reward without dopamine. *The Journal of Neuroscience, 23,* 10827–10831.

Cannon, W. B. (1929). *Bodily changes in pain, hunger fear, and rage.* New York: Appleton.

Cardinal, R. N., Pennicott, D. R., Sugathapala, C. L., Robbins, & T. W., Everitt, B. J. (2001). Impulsive choice induced in rats by lesions of the nucleus accumbens core. *Science, 292,* 2499–2501.

Carey, S. (2004). Bootstrapping and the origins of concepts. *Dcedalus, Winter,* 59–68.

Carlezon, W. A., Jr., & Wise, R. A. (1996). Rewarding actions of phencyclidine and related drugs in nucleus accumbens shell and frontal cortex. *Journal of Neuroscience, 16,* 3112–3122.

Carlson, S. M., Moses, L. J., & Hix, H. R. (1998). The role of inhibitory processes in young children's difficulties with deception and false belief. *Child Development, 69,* 672–691.

Carlsson, A., Hansson, L. O., Waters, N., & Carlsson, M. L. (1997). Neurotransmitter aberrations in schizophrenia: New perspectives and therapeutic implications. *Life Sciences, 61,* 75–94.

Castelli, F., Happe, F., Frith, U., & Frith, C. (2000). Movement and mind: A functional imaging study of perception interpretation of complex intentional movement patterns. *Neuroimage, 12*, 314–325.

Chaminade, T., Meltzoff, A. N., & Decety, J. (2002). Does the end justify the means: A PET exploration of the mechanisms involved in human imitation. *Neuroimage, 15*, 318–328.

Champagne, F. A., Chreiten, P., Stevenson, C. W., Zhang, T. Y., Gratton, A., & Meaneym M. J. (2004). Variations in nucleus accumbens dopamine associated with individual differences in maternal behavior in the rat. *Journal of Neuroscience, 24*, 4113–4123.

Changeux, J-P., & Chyavaillon, J. (Eds.). (1995). *Origins of the human brain*. Oxford, UK: Clarendon Press.

Chomsky, N. (1972). *Language and mind*. New York: Harcourt Press.

Chung, S., & Herrnstein, R. J. (1967). Choice and delay of reinforcement. *Journal of the Experimental Analysis of Behavior, 10*, 67–74.

Churchland, P. S. (2002). *Brain wise*. Cambridge: MIT Press.

Churchland, P. S., & Sejnowski, T. J. (1990). In L. Nadel, L. Cooper, P. Culicover, & M. Harnish (Eds.), *Neural connections, mental computation* (pp.). Cambridge: MIT Press.

Cicero. (1991). *On duties*. New York: Cambridge University Press.

Clark, A. (1999). An Embodied cognitive science. *Trends in Cognitive Science, 3*, 345–351.

Coco, M. L., & Weiss, J. M. (2005). Neural substrates of coping behavior in the rat: possible importance of mesocorticolimbic dopamine system. *Behavioral Neuroscience, 119*(2), 429–445.

Cohen, J. D., & Sevan-Schreiber, D. (1993). A theory of dopamine functions and its role in cognitive deficits in schizophrenia. *Schizophrenia Bulletin, 19*, 85–104.

Cohen, S. B., Robertson, M. M., & Moriarty, J. (1994). The development of the will: A neuropsychological analysis of Gilles de la Tourette Syndrome. In D. Ciccetti & S. Toth (Eds.), *Disorders and dysfunctions of the self*. Rochester Symposium on Developmental Psychopathology (pp. 57–77). Rochester, NY: University of Rochester Press.

Cools, R. (2005). Review: Dopaminergic modulation of cognitive function-implications for L-Dopa treatment in Parkinson's disease. *Neuroscience and Biobehavioral Reviews*, 1–23.

Cools, R., & Robbins, T. W. (2004). Chemistry of the adaptive mind. *Philosophical Transactions of the Royal Society of London, 362*, 2871–2888.

Craig, W. C. (1918). Appetites and aversions as constituents of instincts. *Biological Bulletin, 34*, 96–103.

Critchley, H. D., Mattias, C. J., & Dolan, R. J. (2001). Neural activity in the human brain relating to uncertainty and arousal during anticipation. *Neuron, 29*, 537–545.

Critchley, M., & Critchley, E. A. (1998). *John Hughlings Jackson*. Oxford, UK: Oxford University Press.

Cromwell, H. C., Berridge, K. C., Drago, J., & Levine, M. S. (1998). Action sequencing is impaired in D1A deficient mice. *European Journal of Neuroscience, 10,* 2426–2432.

Cummings, J. L. (1993). Frontal-subcortical circuits and human behavior. *Archives of Neurology, 50,* 873–880.

Damasio, A. (1994). *Descartes' error: Emotion, reason, and the human brain*. New York: Grosset/Putnam.

Damasio, A. (1999). *The feeling of what happens*. New York: Harcourt Press.

Dao-Castellana, M. H., Samson, Y., Legault, F., Martinot, J. L., Aubin, H. J., Crouzel, C., Feldman, L., Barrucand, D., Rancurel, G., Feline, A., & Syrota, A. (1998). Frontal dysfunction in neurologically normal chronic alcoholic subjects: Metabolic and neuropsychological findings. *Psychological Medicine, 28*(5), 1039–1048.

Darwin, C. (1871, 1874). *The descent of man and selection in relation to sex*. Chicago: Rand McNally.

Darwin, C. (1958). *The origin of species*. New York: Mentor Books. (Original work published 1859)

Darwin, C. (1998). *The expression of the emotions in man and animals*. Oxford, UK: Oxford University Press. (Original work published 1872)

Dasser, V., Ulbaek, I., & Premack, D. (1989). The perception of intention. *Science, 243,* 365–367.

Daugherty, T. K., Quay, H. C., & Ramos, L. (1993). Response perseveration, inhibitory control, and central dopaminergic activity in childhood behavior disorders. *Journal of Genetic Psychology, 154,* 177–188.

Davidson, D. (1969). How is weakness of the will possible? In J. Feinberg (Ed.), *Moral concepts* (pp. 93–113). Oxford, UK: Oxford University Press.

Davidson, R. J., Abercrombie, H., Nitschke, J. B., & Putnam, K. (1999). Regional brain function, emotion and disorders of emotion. *Current Opinion in Neurobiology, 9,* 228–234.

Davidson, R. J., Ekman, P., Saron, C. D., Senulis, J. A., & Friesnen, W. V. (1990). Approach-withdrawal and cerebral symmetry: emotional expression and brain physiology. *Journal of Personality and Social Psychology, 2,* 330–341.

Davidson, R. J., & Rickman, M. (1999). Behavioral inhibition and the emotional circuitry of the brain. In L. A. Schmidt & J. Schulkin (Eds.), *Extreme fear, shyness and social phobia* (pp. 67–87). Oxford, UK: Oxford University Press.

Davidson, R. J., Scherer, K. R., & Goldsmith, H. H. (2003). *Handbook of affective neuroscience*. Oxford, UK: Oxford University Press.

Decety, J., Chaminade, T., Grèzes, J., & Meltzoff, A. N., (2002). A PET exploration of the neural mechanisms involved in reciprocal imitation. *Neuroimage, 15*, 265–272.

Decety, J., & Grèzes, J. (1999). Neural mechanisms subserving the perception of human actions. *Trends in Cognitive Science, 3*, 172–178.

Decety, J., Perani, D., & Jeannerod, M., (1997). Brain activity during observation of actions: Influence of action content and subject's strategy. *Brain, 120*, 1763–1777.

Decety, J. et al. (1994). Mapping motor representations with positron emission tomography. *Nature, 371*, 598–602.

Deecke, L. (1996). Planning, preparation, execution, and imagery of volitional action. *Cognitive Brain Research, 3*, 59–64.

Defelipe, J., & Jones, E. G. (1988). *Cajal on the cerebral cortex: An annotated translation of the complete writings*. Oxford, UK: Oxford University Press.

Dennett, D. C. (1984; 1999). *Elbow room: The varieties of free will worth wanting*. Cambridge: MIT Press.

Dennett, D. C. (1987). *The intentional stance*. Cambridge: MIT Press.

Dennett, D. C. (2003). *Freedom evolves*. New York: Viking Press.

Denny-Brown, D. (1951). The frontal lobes and their functions. In A. Feiling (Ed.), *Modern trends in neurology* (pp. 13–89). London: Butterworth.

Denton, D. (1982). *Sodium hunger*. New York: Springer-Verlag.

Depue, R. A., & Morrone-Strupinsky, J. V. (2005). A neurobehavioral model of affiliative bonding: Implications for conceptualizing a human trait of affiliation, *Behavioral and Brain Sciences, 28*, 313–395.

Descombes, V. (2001). *The mind's provisions*. Princeton, NJ: Princeton University Press.

Dethier, V. G. (1982). The contribution of insects to the study of motivation. In A. R. Morrison & P. L. Strick (Eds.), *Changing concepts in the nervous system* (pp. 445–455). New York: Academic Press.

Dewey, J. (1896). The reflex arc concept in psychology. *Psychological Review, 3*, 357–370.

Dewey, J. (1965). *The Influence of Darwin on Philosophy*. Bloomington: Indiana University Press. (Original work published 1910)

Dewey, J. (1975). *The early works, 1882–1898: Vol. 2, 1887, Psychology.* Carbondale: Southern Illinois University Press. (Original work published 1887)

Dewey, J. (1989). *Experience and nature.* Chicago: Open Court. (Original work published 1925)

Diamond, A. (2001). A model system for studying the role of dopamine in the prefrontal cortex during early development in humans: early and continuously treated phenylketonuria. In C.A. Nelson & M. Luciana (Eds.), *Handbook of developmental cognitive neuroscience* (pp. 433–472). Cambridge: MIT Press.

Diamond, A., Goldman-Rakic, P. S. (1989). Comparison of human infants and rhesus monkeys on Piaget's AB task: evidence for dependence on dorsolateral prefrontal cortex. *Experimental Brain Research, 74,* 24–40.

Diamond, A., Prevor, M. B., Callender, G., & Druin, D. P. (1997). Prefrontal cortex cognitive deficits in children treated early and continuously for PKU. *Monographs of the Society for Research in Child Development, 62*(4).

Diaz-Anzaldua, A., Jober, R., Riviere, J. B., Dion, Y., Lesperance, P., Rucgter, F., Chouinard, S., Rouleau, G. A., et al. (2004). Tourette syndrome and dopaminergic genes: A family-based association study in the French Canadian founder population. *Molecular Psychiatry, 9,* 272–277.

Di Chiara, G. (1999). Drug addiction as dopamine-dependent associative learning. *European Journal of Pharmacology, 375,* 13–30.

Di Pellegrino, G., Fadiga, L., Fogassi, L., Gallese, V., & Rizzolatti, G. (1992). Understanding motor events: A neurophysiological study. *Experimental Brain Research, 91,* 176–180.

Dommett, E., Coizet, V., Blaha, C. D., Martindale, J., Lefebvre, V., Walton, N., et al. (2005). How visual stimuli activate dopaminergic neurons at short latency. *Science, 307,* 1476–1479.

Dooley, P. K. (2001). Public policy and the philosophical critique: The William James and T. Roosevelt dialogue on strenuousness. *Journal of C.S. Peirce Society, 35,* 161–169.

Double, R. (1991). *The non-reality of free will.* Oxford, UK: Oxford University Press.

Drabant, E. M.,. Harir, A. R., Munoz, K. E., Kolachana, B. S., Egan, B. S., & Weinbergerm D. R. (2004). Genetic variation in dopamine signaling alters amygdala reactivity. *Neuroscience Abstracts 785.15.*

Dreisbach, G., Muller, J., Goschke, T., Strobel, A., Schulze, K., Lesch, K.-P., et al. (2005). Dopamine and cognitive control: The influence of spontaneous eyeblink rate and dopamine gene polymorphisms on perseration and distractibility. *Behavioral Neuroscience, 119,* 483–490.

Dretske, F. (1994). *Naturalizing the mind.* Cambridge: MIT Press.

Drevets, W. C., Gautier, C., Price, J. C. Kupfer, D. J., Kinahan, P. E., Gracem A. A., et al. (2001). Amphetamine-induced dopamine release in human ventral striatum correlates with euphoria. *Biological Psychiatry, 49,* 49–81.

Dupre, J. (1996). The solution to the problem of the freedom of the will. *Philosophical Perspectives, 10,* 385–402.

Eichenbaum, H., & Cohen, N.J. (2001). *From conditioning to conscious recollection.* Oxford, UK: Oxford University Press.

Eidelberg, D., Moeller, J. R., Antonini, A., Kazumata, K., Dhawan, V., Budman, C., et al. (1997). The metabolic anatomy of Tourette's syndrome. *Neurology, 48,* 927–934.

Elsner, B. & Hommel, B. (2001). Effect anticipation and action control. *Journal of Experiment Psychology, Human Perception and Performance, 27,* 229–240.

Elster, J. (1979). *Ulysses and the sirens: Studies in rationality and irrationality.* Cambridge, UK: Cambridge University Press.

Elster, J. (1999). *Strong feelings.* Cambridge: MIT Press.

Elster, J. (2000). *Ulysses unbound.* Cambridge, UK: Cambridge University Press.

Elster, J., & Skog, O-.J. (1999 Editors): *Getting hooked. Rationality and addiction.* Cambridge, UK: Cambridge University Press.

Epstein, A. N. (1982). Instinct and motivation as explanations for complex behaviour. In D. W. Pfaff (Ed.), *The physiological mechanisms of motivation* (pp. 25–58). New York: Springer.

Erickson K. I. et al. (2003). Behavioral conflict, anterior cingulate cortex and experiment duration: Implications of diverging data. *Human Brain Mapping, 21,* 98–107.

Espejo, E. F. (2003). Prefrontocortical dopamine loss in rats delays long-term extinction of contextual conditioned fear, and reduces social interaction without affecting short-term social interaction memory. *Neuropsychopharmacology, 28,* 490–498.

Evarts, E. V. (1973). Brain mechanisms in movement. *Scientific American, 229*(1), 96–103.

Evarts, E. V. (1981). Role of motor cortex in voluntary movements in primates. In V. B. Brooks (Ed.), *Handbook of physiology* (pp. 48–70). Bethesda, MD: American Physiological Society.

Everitt, B. J., & Robbins, T. W. (2005). Neural systems of reinforcement for drug addiction: From actions to habits to compulsions. *Nature Neuroscience, 11,* 1481–1489.

Fanselow, M. S. (1994). Neural organization of the defensive behavior system responsible for fear. *Psychonomic Bulletin and Review, 1,* 429–438.

Farrer, C., & Frith, C. D. (2002). Experiencing oneself vs another person as being the cause of an action: The neural correlates of the experience of agency. *Neuroimage, 15,* 596–603.

Fehling C. (1966). Treatment of Parkinson's disease with L-DOPA: Double blind study. *Acta Neurologica Scandinavica, 42,* 367–372.

Fentress, J. C. (1982). Ethological models of hierarchy and patterning of species specific behavior. In E. Satinoff & P. Teitelbaum (Eds.), *Handbook of behavioral neurobiology* (Vol. 6, pp. 185–234). New York: Plenum Press.

Ferrier, D. (1886). *The functions of the brain* (2nd ed.). London: Smith, Elder.

Finger, S. (1994). *Origins of neuroscience.* New York: Oxford University Press.

Finger, S. (2000). *Minds behind the brain.* New York: Oxford University Press.

Fitzsimons, J. T. (1998). Angiotensin, thirst, and sodium appetite. *Physiological Review, 78,* 583–686.

Flanagan, O. J. (1984). *The science of mind.* Cambridge: MIT Press.

Florillo, C. D., Tobler, P. N., & Schultz, W. (2003). Discrete coding of reward probability and uncertainty by dopamine neurons. *Science, 299,* 1989–1991.

Flourens, M. J. P. (1824). Recherches expérimentales sur les propriétés et les fonctions du systèmes nerveux dans les animaux vertébrés. Paris: J. B. Balliere.

Fluharty, S. J. (2002). Neuroendocrinology of body fluid homeostasis. In D. Pfaff (Ed.), *Hormones, brain and behavior* (pp. 1010–1025). New York: Academic Press.

Flynn, J. P. (1972). Patterning mechanisms, patterned reflexes, and attack behavior in cats. *Nebraska Symposium on Motivation, 20,* 125–153.

Fowler, J. S., Volkow, N. D., Malison, R., & Gatley, S. J. (1999). Neuroimaging studies of substance abuse disorders. In D. S. Charney, E. J. Nestler, & B. S. Bunney (Eds.), *Neurobiology of mental illness.* New York: Oxford University Press.

Frankfurt, H. G. (1971). Freedom of will and the concept of a person. *Journal of Philosophy, 68,* 5–20.

Frankfurt, H. G. (1988). *The importance of what we care about.* Cambridge, UK: Cambridge University Press.

Frankmann, S. P., Broder, L., Dokko, J. H., & Smith, G. P. (1994). Differential changes in central monoaminergic metabolism during first and multiple sodium depletions in rats. *Pharmacology, Biochemistry and Behavior, 47,* 617–624.

Frese, M., & Sabini, J. (1985). *Goal directed behavior.* Hillsdale, NJ: Lawrence Erlbaum Associates.

Freud, S. (1959). Inhibitions, symptoms and anxiety (A. Strachey, Trans., J. Strachey, Ed.). New York: Norton. (Original work published 1926)

Freud, S. (1966). Project for a scientific psychology. In E. Jones (Ed.) & J. Strachey (Trans.), The standard edition of the complete psychological works of Sigmund Freud (Vol. 1, pp. 295–387). (Unpublished manuscript written 1895)

Fried, I., Wilson, C. L., Morrow J. W., Cameron, K. A. Behnke, E. D., Ackerson, L. C., et al. (2001). Increased dopamine release in the human amygdala during performance of cognitive tasks. Nature Neuroscience, 4, 201–206.

Frijda, N. (1986). The emotions. Cambridge, UK: Cambridge University Press.

Frith, C. D. (1992). The cognitive neuropsychology of schizophrenia. Hillsdale, NJ: Lawrence Erlbaum Associates.

Frith, C. D., Friston, K., Liddle, P. F., & Frackowiak, R. S. J. (1991). Willed action and the prefrontal cortex in man: A study with PET. Proceedings of the Royal Society of London, B244, 241–246.

Frith, C. D., and Frith, U. (1999). Interacting minds—biological basis. Science, 286: 1692–1695.

Fruend, H. J. (1990). Premotor area and preparation of movement. Review of Neurology, 146, 543–547.

Fulton, J. F. (1949). Functional localization in the frontal lobes and cerebellum. Oxford, UK: Oxford University Press.

Fuster, J. M. (1997). The prefrontal cortex: Anatomy, physiology, and neuropsychology of the frontal lobe (3rd ed.). Philadelphia: Lippincott-Raven.

Fuster, J. M. (2001). The prefrontal cortex—An update: Time is of the essence. Neuron, 30, 319–333.

Gallese, V., Fadiga, L., Fogassi, F. & Rizzolatti, G. (1996). Action recognition in the premotor cortex. Brain, 119, 593–609.

Gallistel, C. R. (1980). The organization of action: A new synthesis. Hillsdale, NJ: Lawrence Erlbaum Associates.

Gallistel, C. R. (1992). The organization of learning. Cambridge: MIT Press.

Gallup, G. G., Jr. (1977). Tonic immobility: The role of fear and predation. The Psychological Record. 1, 41–61.

Garavan, H., Ross, T. J., & Stein, E. A. (1999). Right hemispheric dominance of inhibitory control: An event-related functional MRI study. Proceedings of the National Academy of Science USA, 96(14), 8301–8306.

Gazzaniga, M. S. (2000). The new cognitive neurosciences (2nd ed.). Cambridge: MIT Press.

Gehring, W. J., & Fenesik, D. E. (2001). Functions of the medial frontal cortex in the processing of conflict and errors. *Journal of Neuroscience, 21*, 9430–9437.

Georgopoulos, A. P. (1994). New concepts in generation of movement. *Neuron, 13*, 257–268.

Georgopoulos, A. P. (2000). Neural mechanisms of motor cognitive processes: functional MRI and neurophysiological studies. In M. S. Gazzaniga (Ed.), *The new cognitive neurosciences* (2nd ed.). Cambridge: MIT Press.

Gigerenzer, G. (2000). *Adaptive thinking, rationality in the real world*. New York: Oxford University Press.

Giles de la Tourette, G. (1885). Etude sur une affection nerveuse caractérisée par de l'incoordination motrice accompagnee d'echolalie et de copralalie. *Archives de Neurologie, 9*, 19–42, 158–200.

Glickman, S. E., & Schiff, B. B. (1967). A biological theory of reinforcement. *Psychological Review, 74*, 81–109.

Glimcher, P. W. (2003). *Decisions, uncertainty and the brain*. Cambridge: MIT Press.

Glimcher, P. W., & Rustichini, A. (2004). Neuroeconomics: The consilience of brain and decision. *Science, 306*, 447–452.

Glynn, I. (1999). *An anatomy of thought*. Oxford, UK: Oxford University Press.

Goldman, A. I. (1970). *A theory of human action*. Englewood Cliffs, NJ: Prentice Hall.

Goldman, A. I. (1990). Action and free will. In D. N. Osherson, S. M. Kosslyhn, & J. M. Hollerbach (Eds.), *Visual cognition and action. An invitation to cognitive science*, (Vol. 2, pp.). Cambridge: MIT Press.

Goldman, P. S., & Nauta, W. J. H. (1977). Columnar distribution of cortico-cortical fibers in the frontal association, limbic and motor cortex of the developing rhesus monkey. *Brain Research, 122*, 393–413.

Goldman, P. S., Rosvold, E., & Mishkin, M. (1970). Evidence for behavioral impairment following prefrontal lobectomy in the infant monkey. *Journal of Comparative and Physiological Psychology, 70*, 454–463.

Goldman-Rakic, P. S. (1987). Circuitry of primate prefrontal cortex and regulation of behavior by representational memory. In V. B. Mountcastle & F. Plum (Eds.), *Handbook of physiology, Section 1. The nervous system: Vol. 5. Higher functions of the brain* (Pt. 1, pp. 373–417). Bethesda, MD: American Physiological Society.

Goldman-Rakic, P. S. (1990). Cellular and circuit basis of working memory in prefrontal areas of non-human primates. *Progress in Brain Research, 85*, 325–336.

Goldman-Rakic, P. S. (1999). The physiological approach: Functional architecture of working memory and disordered cognition in schizophrenia. *Biological Psychiatry, 46,* 650–661.

Goldman-Rakic, P. S., Leranth, C., Williams, S. M., Mons, N., & Gerrard, M. (1989). Dopamine synaptic complex with pyradidal neurons in primate cerebral cortex. *Proceedings of the National Academy of Sciences, 86,* 9015–9019.

Goldstein, K. (1939). *The organism. A holistic approach to biology derived from pathological data in man.* New York: American Book.

Goldstein, K. (1944). The mental changes due to frontal lobe damage. *Journal of Psychology, 17,* 187–208.

Gollwitzer, P. M. (1996). The volitional benefits of planning. In P. M. Gollwitzer, & J. A. Bargh (Eds.), *The psychology of action: Linking cognition and motivation to behavior* (pp. 287–312). New York: Guilford Press.

Gould, S. J. (2002). *The structure of evolutionary theory.* Cambridge, MA: Harvard University Press.

Grant, S., London, E. D., Newlin, D. B., Villemagne, V. L., Liu, X., Contoreggi, C., Phillips, R. L., Kimes, A. S., & Margolin, A. (1996). Activation of memory circuits during cue-elicited cocaine cravings. *Proceedings of the National Academy of Sciences, USA, 93*(21), 12040–12045.

Gray, J. A. (1971). *The psychology of fear and stress.* London: Weidenfeld & Nicolson.

Graybiel, A. M. (2001). Neural networks: Neural systems V: Basal ganglia. *American Journal of Psychiatry, 158,* 21–27.

Graybiel, A. M., Aosaki, T., Flaherty, A. W., & Kimura, M. (1994). The basal ganglia and adaptive motor control. *Science, 265,* 1826–1931.

Graybiel, A. M., Moratalla, R., & Robertso, H. A. (1990). Amphetamine and cocaine induce drug-specific activation of the c-fos gene in striosome-matrix compartments and limbic subdivisions of the striatum. *Proceedings of the National Academy of Sciences, 87,* 6912–6916.

Greenberg, B. D. (1997). The role of neurotransmitters and neurohormones in obsessive-compulsive disorder. *International Review of Psychiatry, 9,* 31–34.

Greenberg, B. D., George, M. S., Mart, J. D., Benjamin, J. et al. (1997). Effect of prefrontal repetitive transcranial magnetic stimulation in obsessive-compulsive disorder: a preliminary study. *American Journal of Psychiatry 154*(6), 867–869.

Greenberg, B. D., Ziemann, U., Cora-Locatelli, G., Harmon, A., Murphy, D. L., Keel, J. C., et al. (2000). Altered cortical excitability in obsessive-compulsive disorder. *Neurology, 54*(1), 142–147.

Greene, J. D., Sommerville, R. B., Nystrom, L. E., Cohen, J. D. (2001). An fMRI investigation of emotional engagement in moral judgement. *Science, 293,* 517–523.

Gross, C. G. (1999). *Brain vision memory. Tales in the history of neuroscience.* Cambridge: MIT Press.

Grossberg, S. (2000). How hallucinations may arise from brain mechanisms of learning, attention, and volition. *Journal of the International Neuropsychological Society, 6,* 583–592.

Hacking, I. (1979). *Logic of statistical inference.* Cambridge, UK: Cambridge University Press. (Original work published 1965)

Hacking, I. (1990). *The taming of chance.* Cambridge, UK: Cambridge University Press.

Haggard, P., Cark, S., & Kalogeras, J. (2002). Voluntary action and conscious awareness. *Nature Neuroscience, 5*(4), 382–385.

Hansen, E. S., Hasselbalch, S., Lay, I., & Bolwig, T. G. (2002). The caudate nucleus in obsessive-compulsive disorder. Reduced metabolism following treatment with paroxetine: A PET study. *International Journal of Neuropharmacology, 5,* 1–10.

Hari, R., Forss, N., Avikainen, S., Kirveskari, E., Salenius, S., & Rizzolatti, G. (1988). Activation of human primary motor cortex during action and observation: A neurmagnetic study. *Proceedings of the National Academy of Science, 95,* 15061–15065.

Hauk, G., Johnsrude, I., & Pulvermuller, F. (2004). Somatotrophic representation of action words in human motor and premotor cortex. *Neuron, 41,* 301–307.

Hebb, D. O. (1949). *The organization of behavior.* New York: Wiley.

Heelan, P. A., & Schulkin, J. (1998). Hermeneutical philosophy and pragmatism: A philosophy of science. *Synthese, 115,* 260–302.

Heidegger, M. (1979). *Nietzsche: Vol. 1. The will to power as art.* (D. F. Krell, Trans.). San Francisco: Harper & Row.

Heimer, L., Switzer, R. D., & Van Hoesen, G. W. (1992). Ventral striatum and ventral pallidum: Components of the motor system? *Trends in Neural Science, 5,* 83–87.

Heinrichs, R. W. (2001). *In search of madness. Schizophrenia and neuroscience.* New York: Oxford University Press.

Herbert, J. (1993). Peptides in the limbic system: Neurochemical codes for co-ordinated adaptive responses to behavioral and physiological demand. *Progress in Neurobiology, 41,* 723–791.

Herbert, J., & Schulkin, J. (2002). Neurochemical coding of adaptive responses in the limbic system. In D. W. Pfaff: (Ed.), *Hormones, brain and behavior* (pp. 617–632). New York: Elsevier.

Hernstein, R. (1997). *The matching law.* Cambridge, MA: Harvard University Press.

Herrnstein, R., & Prelec, D. (1992). A theory of addiction. In G. Loewenstein & J. Elster (Eds.), *Choice over time* (pp. 331–360). New York: Russell Sage Foundation.

Hinde, R. A. (1970). *Animal behavior* (2nd ed.). New York: McGraw-Hill.

Hirschman, A. O. (1981). *The passions and the interests.* Princeton, NJ: Princeton University Press.

Hitzig, E. (1900). Hughlings Jackson and the cortical motor centres in the light of physiological research. *Brain, 23,* 545–581.

Hoebel, B. G. (1988). Neuroscience of motivation: Peptides and pathways that define motivational systems. In S. S. Stevens (Ed.), *Handbook of experimental psychology.* New York: Wiley.

Hoebel, B. G. (1998). Neural systems for reinforcement and inhibition of behavior: Relevance to eating, addiction and depression. In D. Kahneman, E. Diener, & N. Schwartz (Eds.), *Understanding quality of life: Scientific perspectives on enjoyment and suffering.*

Hollander, E., DeCaria, K. M., Schneier, F. R., Schneier, H. A., Liebowitz, M. R., & Klein, D. F. (1990). Fenfluramine augmentation of serotonin reuptake blockade antiobsessional treatment. *Journal of Clinical Psychiatry, 51,* 119–122.

Hollerman, J. R., Tremblay, L., & Schultz, W. (2000). Involvement of basal ganglia and orbitofrontal cortex in goal-directed behavior. *Progress in Brain Research, 126,* 193–215.

Holloway, R. L. (1995). Toward a synthetic theory of human brain evolution. In J.-P. Changeux & J. Chavaillon (Eds.), *Origins of the human brain* (pp.). Oxford, UK: Clarendon Press.

Holst, E. von (1973). Relative coordination as a phenomenon and as a method of analysis of central nervous functions. In *The behavioral physiology of animals and man. Selected papers of Eric von Holst.* Coral Gables, FL: University of Miami Press.

Hommel, B. (1996). The cognitive representation of action: automatic integration of perceived action effects. *Psychological Research, 59,* 176–186.

Honderich, T. (2002). How free are you (2nd ed.). Oxford, UK: Oxford University Press.

Horsley, V. (1909). The function of the so-called "motor" area of the brain. *British Medical Journal, 21,* 125–132.

Horvitz, J. C. (2000). Meolimbicortical and nigrostriatal dopamine responses to salient non-reward events. *Neuroscience, 96,* 651–656.

Howard, M. O., Kivlahan, D., & Walker, R. D. (1997). Cloninger's tridimensional theory of personality and psychopathology: Applications to substance use disorders. *Journal of Studies on Alcoholism, 58*(1), 48–66.

Hume, D. (1964). *A Treatise of Human Nature* (L. A. Selvy-Bigge, Ed.). Oxford, UK: Clarendon. (Original work published 1739)

Humphrey, D. R., & Freund, H. J. (1991). *Motor control*. New York: Wiley.

Ikemoto, S., & Panksepp, J. (1999). The role of nucleus accumbens dopamine in motivated behavior: A unifying interpretation with special reference to reward-seeking. *Brain Research Reviews, 31*, 6–41.

Ingvar, D. H. (1994). The will of the brain: Cerebral correlates of willful acts. *Journal of Theoretical Biology, 171*, 7–12.

Insel, T. R. (1992). Toward a neuroanatomy of obsessive-compulsive disorder. *Archives of General Psychiatry, 49*, 739–744.

Insel, T. R., Mueller, E. A., Alterman, I., Linnoila, M., & Murphy, D. L. (1985). Obsessive-compulsive disorder and serotonin: Is there a connection? *Biological Psychiatry, 20*, 1174–1188.

Isomura, Y., Ito, Y., Akazawa, T., Nambu, A., & Takada, M. (2003). Neural coding of attention for action and response selection in primate anterior cingulate cortex. *Journal of Neuroscience, 23*, 8002–8112.

Iversen, S. D., & Mishkin, M. (1970). Perseverative interference in monkeys following selective lesions of the inferior prefrontal convexity. *Exp. Brain Res. 11*(4): 376–386.

Jabre, J. F., & Salzsieder, B. T. (1997). The volitional unit: a functional concept I cortico-motoneuronal connections in humans. *Electroncephalography and clinical Neurophysiology, 105*, 365–369.

Jackson, J. H. (1863). Convulsive spasms of the right hand and arm preceding epileptic seizures. *Medical Times and Gazette, 1*, 110–111.

Jackson, J. H. (1958). On some implications of dissolution of the nervous system. In J. Taylor (Ed.), Selected writings of John Hughlings Jackson. London: Staples Press. (Original work published 1882)

Jackson, P. L., & Decety, J. (2004). Motor cognition: A new paradigm to self and other interactions. *Current Opinion in Neurobiology, 14*, 259–263.

Jacob, P., & Jeannerod, M. (2003). *Ways of seeing*. Oxford, UK: Oxford University Press.

James, W. (1952). *The principles of psychology* (Vols. 1 & 2). New York: Dover. (Original work published 1890)

James, W. (1897). The will to believe. In W. James (Ed.), *The will to believe and other essays in popular philosophy* (pp. 1–31). New York: Longmans, Green.

James, W. (1958). *Talks to teachers on psychology: And to students on some of life's ideals*. New York: Norton. (Original work published 1899)

Janet, J. (1906). On the pathogenesis of some impulsions. *Journal of Abnormal Psychology, 1,* 1–17.

Jang, K. L., Livesley, W. J., & Vernon, P. A. (1997). Gender-specific etiological differences in alcohol and drug problems: A Behavioral genetic analysis. *Addiction 92*(10), 1265–1276.

Jaspers, K. (1997). *General psychopathology, Vols 1 and 2.* (J. Hoenig & M. W. Hamilton, Trans.). Baltimore: Johns Hopkins University Press. (Original work published 1913)

Jeannerod, M. (1985). *The brain machine.* Cambridge, MA: Harvard University Press.

Jeannerod, M. (1988). *The neural and behavioral organization of goal-directed movements.* Oxford, UK: Clarendon Press.

Jeannerod, M. (1994). The representing brain: Neural correlates of motor intention and imagery. *Behavioral Brain Science, 17,* 187–245.

Jennings, J. R., van der Molen, M. W., Pelham, W., Debski, K. B., & Hoza, B. (1997). Inhibition in boys with attention deficit hyperactivity disorder as indexed by heart rate change. *Developmental Psychology, 33*(2), 308–318.

Kagan, J. (1999). The concept of behavioral inhibition. In L. A. Schmidt & J. Schulkin (Eds.), *Extreme fear, shyness, and social phobia.* New York: Oxford University Press.

Kagan, J. (2002). *Surprise, uncertainty and mental structure.* Cambridge, MA: Harvard University Press.

Kagan, J., Kearsley, R. B., & Zelazo, P. R. (1980). *Infancy.* Cambridge, MA: Harvard University Press.

Kagan, J., Resnick, J. S., & Snidman, N. (1988). Biological basis of childhood shyness. *Science, 240,* 167–171.

Kagan, J., & Schulkin, J. (1995). On the concepts of fear. *Harvard Review of Psychiatry, 3,* 31–34.

Kahneman, D., Diener, E., & Schwarz, N. (1999). *Well-being: The foundations of hedonic psychology.* New York: Russell Sage Foundation.

Kahneman, D., Slovic, P., & Tversky, A. (Eds.). (1982). *Judgment under uncertainty; Heuristics and biases.* Chapter 1 originally appeared in Science, 1974, 185, 1124–1131. Cambridge: Cambridge University Press.

Kaiser, J., Barker, R., Haensche, C., Baldeweg, T., & Gruzeller, J. H. (1997). Hypnosis and event-related potential correlates of error processing in a stroop-type paradigm: A test of the frontal hypothesis. *International Journal of Psychophysiology, 27*(3), 215–222.

Kallio, S., Revonsuo, A., Hamalainen, H., Markela, J., & Gruzelier, J. (2001). Anterior brain functions and hypnosis: A test of the frontal hypothesis. *International Journal of Clinical & Experimental Hypnosis, 49*(2), 95–108.

Kandel, E. R., & Squire, L. R. (2000). Neuroscience: Breaking down scientific barriers to the study of brain and mind. *Science, 290,* 1113–1120.

Kane, R. (1995). Jamesian reflections on will, freedom, and value. In R. Burch (Ed.), *Frontiers in American philosophy* (Vol. 2, pp. 365–374). College Station: Texas A&M University Press.

Kane, R. (1998). *The significance of free will.* New York: Oxford University Press.

Kane, R. (2002). *The handbook of free will.* Oxford, UK: University Press.

Kapp, B. S., Frysinger, R. C., Gallaher, M., & Haselton, J. (1979). Amygdala central nucleus lesions: Effect on heart rate conditioning in the rabbit. *Physiology and Behavior, 23,* 1109–1117.

Kelley, A. E. (1999). Neural integrative activities of nucleus accumbens subregions in relation to learning and motivation. *Psychobiology, 27*(2), 198–213.

Kelley, A. E. (2004). Ventral striatal control of appetitive motivation: Role in ingestive behavior and reward-related learning. *Neuroscience and Biobehavioral Reviews, 27,* 765–776.

Kelley, A. E., Domesick, V. B., & Nauta, W. J. H. (1982). The amygdalostriatal projection in the rat: An anatomical study by anterograde and retrograde tracing methods. *Neuroscience, 7,* 615–630.

Kenny, A. (1976). *Action, emotion and will.* London: Routledge & Kegan Paul.

Kerns, J. G., Cohen, J. D., MacDonald, A. W., Cho, R. Y., Stenger, V. A., & Carter, C. S. (2004). Anterior cingulate conflict monitoring and adjustments in control. *Science, 202,* 1023–1026.

Kimura, D. (1993). *Neuromotor mechanism in human communication.* Oxford, UK: Oxford University Press.

Kirby, K. N. (1997). Bidding on the future: Evidence against normative discounting of delayed rewards. *Journal of Experimental Psychology: General, 126,* 54–70.

Kirley, A. (2002). Dopaminergic system genes in ADHD: Toward a biological hypothesis. *Neuropharmacology, 27,* 607–619.

Kish, S. J., Kalasinsky, K. S., Derkach, P., et al. (2001). Striatal dopaminergic and serotinergic markers in human heroin users. *Neuropharmacology, 24,* 561–567.

Knowlton, B., Mangels, J., & Squire, L. (1996). A neostriatal habit learning system in humans. *Science, 273,* 1399–1402.

Kohler, E., Keysers, C., Umilta, M. A., Fogassi, L., Gallese, V., & Rizzolatti, G. (2002). Hearing sounds, understanding actions: action representation in mirror neurons. *Science, 297,* 846–848.

Konishi, S., Nakajima, K., Uchida, I., Kikyo, H., Kameyama, M., & Miyashita, Y. (1999). Common inhibitory mechanism in human inferior prefrontal cortex revealed by event-related functional MRI. *Brain, 122*(Pt5), 981–991.

Konorski, J. (1967). *Integrative activity of the brain*. Chicago: University of Chicago Press.

Koob, G. F. (1998). The role of the striatopallidal and extended amygdala systems in drug addiction. *Annals of the New York Academy of Sciences, 877*, 445–460.

Koob, G. F., & LeMoal, M. (2001). Drug addiction, dysregulation of reward, and allostasis. *Neuropsychopharmacology, 24*, 94–129.

Koob, G. F., & LeMoal, M. (2005). *Neurobiology of addiction*. New York: Elsevier.

Kosslyn, S. (1994). *Image and brain*. Cambridge: MIT Press.

Korpi, E. R., Kleinman, J. E., Goodman, S. I., & Wyatt, R. J. (1987). Neurotransmitter amino acids in post-mortem brains of chronic schizophrenic patients. *Psychiatry Research, 22*, 291–301.

Kraepelin, E. (1919). Dementia praecox and paraphrenia (R. M. Barclay, Trans., G. M. Robertson, Ed.), (pp.1–331), Edinburgh: E & S Livingstone.

Kraines, S. H. (1969). Hypnosis: physiologic inhibition and excitation. *Behavioral Neuropsychiatry. 1*(6), 11–16.

Krause, K. H., Dresel, S. H., Krause, J., Foungere, C., & Ackenheil, M. (2003). The dopamine transporter and neuroimaging in attention deficit hyperactivity disorder. *Neuroscience and Biobehavioral Reviews, 27*, 605–613.

Kreek, M. J., Nielsen, D. A., Butelman, E. R., & Laforge, S. (2005). Genetic influences on impulsivity, drug abuse and addiction. *Nature Neuroscience, 8*, 1450–1457.

Krieckhaus, E. E., Donahoe, J. W., & Morgan, M. A. (1992). Paranoid schizophrenia may be caused by dopamine hyperactivity of CA1 hippocampus. *Biological Psychiatry, 31*(6), 560–570.

Krieckhaus, E. E., & Wolf, G. (1968). Acquisition of sodium by rats: Interaction of innate mechanisms and latent learning. *Journal of Comparative and Physiological Psychology, 65*, 197–201.

Lakoff, G. (1987). *Women, fire and dangerous things: What categories recalibrate the mind*. Chicago: Chicago University Press.

Lakoff, G., & Johnson, M. (1999). *Philosophy in the flesh*. New York: Basic Books.

Lamarck, J. B. (1984). *Zoological philosophy* (H. Elliott, Trans.). Chicago: University of Chicago Press. (Original work published 1809)

Lashley, K. S. (1938). An experimental analysis of instinctive behavior. *Psychological Review, 45*, 445–471.

Lashley, K. S. (1951). The problem of serial order in behavior. In L.A. Jeffres (Ed.) *Cerebral mechanisms in behavior* (pp. 110–133). New York: Wiley.

Laviotte, S. R., Nader, K., & Vander Kooy, D. (2002). Motivational state determines the functional role of the mesolimbic dopamine system in the mediation of opiate reward processes. *Behavioral Brain Research 129*, 17–29.

Leckman, J. F., Goodman, W. K., Anderson, G. M., Riddle, M. A., Chappell, P. B., McSwiggan-Hardin, M. T., et al. (1995). Cerebrospinal fluid biogenic amines in obsessive compulsive disorder, Tourette's syndrome and healthy controls. *Neuropsychopharmacology, 12*(1), 73–86.

Leckman, J. F., Peterson, B. S., Anderson, G. M., Arnsten, A. F. T., Pauls, D. L., & Cohen, D. J. (1997). Pathogenesis of Tourette's syndrome. *Journal of Child Psychology and Psychiatry, 38*, 119–142.

LeDoux, J. (1996). *The emotional brain: The mysterious underpinnings of emotional life*. New York: Simon & Schuster.

LeDoux, J. E. (2000). Emotion circuits in the brain. *Annual Review of Neuroscience, 23*, 155–184.

LeVasseur, A. L., Flanagan, J. R., Riopelle, R. J., & Munoz, D. P. (2001). Control of volitional and reflexive saccades in Tourette's syndrome. *Brain, 124*, 2045–2058.

Leyton, M., Boileau, I., Benkelfat, C., Diksic, M., Baker, G., & Dagher, A. (2002). Amphetamine-induced increases in extracellular dopamine, drug wanting and novelty seeking: a PET study in healthy men. *Neuropharmacology, 27*, 1027–1035.

Libet, B. (1985). Are the mental experiences of will and self-control significant for the performance of a voluntary act? *Behavioral and Brain Sciences, 10*, 783–791.

Libet, B. (2004). *Mind time*. Cambridge, MA: Harvard University Press.

Lichtheim, L. (1885). On aphasia. *Brain, 7*, 433–484.

Liddle, P. F. (1994). Volition and schizophrenia. In A. S. David & J. C. Cutting (Eds.), *The neuropsychology of schizophrenia* (pp. 39–49). Hove, UK: Erlbaum.

Liddle, P., Kiehl, K., & Smith, A. (2001). Event-related fMRI study of response inhibition. *Human Brain Mapping, 12*, 100–109.

Lieberman, P. (2000). *Human language and our reptilian brain: The subcortical bases of speech, syntax, and thought*. Cambridge: Harvard University Press.

Lim, M. M., Wang, X., Olazabal, D. E., Ren, X., Terwilliger, E. F., & Young, L. J. (2004). Enhanced partner preference in a promiscuous species by manipulating the expression of a single gene. *Nature, 429*, 754–757.

Linas, R. R. (2001). *I of the vortex: From neurons to self.* Cambridge: MIT Press.

Lindley, S. E., Bengoechea, T. G., Schatzberg, A. F., & Wong, D. L. (1999). Glucocorticoid effects on mesotelencephalic dopamine neurotransmission. *Neuropharmacology, 21,* 399–407.

Loewenstein, G. F. (1996). Out of control: Visceral influences on behavior. *Organizational Behavior and Human Decision Processes, 35,* 272–292.

Loewenstein, G. F. (1999). A visceral account of addiction. In J. Elster & O. J. Skog (Eds.), *Getting hooked: Rationality and addiction.* Cambridge, UK: Cambridge University Press.

Loewenstein, G. F., & Schkade, D. (1998). Wouldn't it be nice? Predicting future feelings. In D. Kahneman, E. E. Diener, & N. Schwartz (Eds.). *Understanding quality of life: Scientific perspectives on enjoyment and suffering.* New York: Russell Sage Foundation.

Logan, D. L., Schachar, R. J., & Tannock, R., (1997). Impulsivity and inhibitory control. *Psychological Science, 8*(1), 60–64.

Lorenz, K. (1965). *Evolution and modification of behavior.* Chicago: University of Chicago Press.

Lorenz, K. (1981). *The foundations of ethology.* New York: Springer.

Lotze, R. H. (1852). Medizinische Psychologie oder Physiologie der Seele. Leipsic, Germany.

Lucas, L. R., Grillo, C. A., & McEwen, B. S. (2003). Involvement of mesolimbic structures in short-term sodium depletion: in situ hybridization and ligand-binding analyses. *Neuroendocrinology, 77,* 408–415.

Lucas, L. R., Pompei, P., & McEwen, B. S. (2000). Salt appetite in salt-replete rats: involvement of mesolimbic structures in deoxycorticosterone-induced salt craving behavior. *Neuroendocrinology, 71,* 386–395.

Luetkenhaus, P., & Bullock, M. (1991). The development of volitional skills. In M. Bullock (Ed.) The development of intentional action: Cognitive, motivational, and interactive processes. Contributions to human development 222, 14–23. Basel, Switzerland: S. Karger.

Luria, A. R. (1966). *Higher cortical functions in man.* New York: Basic Books.

Luria, A. R. (1976). *The nature of human conflicts: Emotion conflict and will.* New York:

Maas, L. C., Lukas, S. E., Kaufman, M. J., Weiss, R. D., Daniels, S. L., Rogers, V. W., Kukes, T. J., & Renshaw, P. F. (1998). Functional magnetic resonance imaging of human brain activation during cue-induced cocaine craving. *American Journal of Psychiatry,* *155*(1), 124–126.

MacLean, P. D. (1978). Effects of lesions of globus pallidus on species-typical display behavior of squirrel monkeys. *Brain Research, 149,* 175–196.

Macmillan, M. B. (1992). Inhibition and the control of behavior: From Gall to Freud via Phineas Gage and the frontal lobes. *Brain and Cognition 19,* 72–104.

Macmillan, M. B. (2000). *An Odd Kind of Fame, Stories of Phineas Gage.* Cambridge: Bradford Book, MIT Press.

Maess, B., Koelsch, S., Gunger, T. C., & Friederici, A. D. (2001). Musical syntax is processed in Broca's area: an MEG study. *Nature Neuroscience, 4*(5), 540–545.

Maquet, P., Faymonville, M. E., Degueldre, C., Delfiore, G., Granck, G., Luxen, A., et al. (1999). Functional neuroanatomy of hypnotic state. *Biological Psychiatry, 45*(3), 327–333.

Marler, P. R., & Hamilton, W. J., III (1966). *Mechanisms of animal behavior.* New York: Wiley.

Marsden, C. D., Merton, H. B., Adam, J. E. R., & Hallett, H. (1978). Automatic and voluntary responses to muscle stretch in man. In J. E. Desmedt (Ed.), *Cerebral motor control in man: Long loop mechanisms* (pp. 167–177). Karger, Basel: Progress in Clinical Neurophysiology.

Marsden, C. D., & Obeso, J. A. (1994). The functions of the basal ganglia and the paradox of stereotaxic surgery in Parkinson's disease. *Brain, 117,* 877–897.

Marshall, J. F., Richardson, J. S., & Teitelbaum, P. (!974). Nigrostriatal bundle damage and the lateral hypothalamic syndrome. *Journal of Comparative and Physiological Psychology, 87,* 808–830.

Marshall, J. F., Turner, B. M., & Teitelbaum, P. (1971). Sensory neglect produced by lateral hypothalamic damage. *Science, 174,* 523–525.

Martin, A., & Chao, L. L. (2001). Semantic memory and the brain: structure and processes. *Current Opinion Neurobiology, 11,* 194–201.

Martin, A., Wiggs, C. L., Ungerleider, L. G., & Haxby, J. V. (1996). Neural correlates of category specific knowledge. *Nature, 379,* 649–652.

Masse, L. C., & Tremblay, R. E. (1997). Behavior of boys in kindergarten and the onset of substance use during adolescence. *Archives of General Psychiatry, 54*(1), 62–68.

Matsumoto, K., & Tanska (2004). Conflict and cognitive control. *Science, 303,* 969–970.

Mayr, E. (1982). *The growth of biological thought.* Cambridge, MA: Harvard University Press.

McClure, S. M., Laibson, D. I., Loewenstein, G., & Cohen, J. D. (2004). Separate neural systems value immediate and delayed monetary rewards. *Science, 306*, 503–506.

McCulloch, W. S., & Pitts, W. (1943). A logical calculus of the ideas immanent in nervous activity. *Bull. of Math. Biol., 5*, 115–133.

McGinn, C. (1997). *Minds and Bodies*. Oxford: Oxford University Press.

McGinn, C. (1999). *The Mysterious Flame*. New York: Basic Books.

McEwen, B. S., & Stellar, E. (1993). Stress and the individual. *Archives Internal Medicine 153*, 2093–2101.

Meaney, M. J., Brake, W., & Gratton, A. (2002). Environmental regulation of the development of mesolimbic dopamine systems. *Psychoneuroendocrinology, 27*, 127–138.

Merikangas, K. R. (1990). The genetic epidemiology of alcoholism. *Psychological Medicine, 20*, 11–22.

Merikangas, K. R., Rounsaville, B. J., & Prusoff, B. A. (1992). Familial factors in vulnerability to substance abuse. In M. Glantz & R. Pickens (Eds.), *Vulnerability to drug abuse*. American Psychiatric Press: Washington, D.C.

Mesulam, M. M. (1998). From sensation to cognition. *Brain, 121*, 1013–1052.

Miller, G. A., Galanter, E., & Pribram, K. H. (1960). *Plans and the Structure of Behavior*. New York: Holt, Rinehart and Winston.

Miller, N. E. (1948). Studies of fear as an acquirable drive: 1. Fear as motivation and fear reduction as reinforcement in the learning of new responses. *Journal of Experimental Psychology, 38*, 89–101.

Miller, N. E. (1959). Liberalization of basic S-R concepts: Extensions to conflict behaviour, motivation and social learning. In S. Koch (Ed.), Psychology: A study of a science (Vol. 2, pp. 196–292). New York: McGraw-Hill.

Milner, B. (1982). Some cognitive effects of frontal-lobe lesions in man. *Philosophical Transactions of the Royal Society, London, 298 (suppl. B)*, 211–226.

Milner, B., Corsi, P. & Leonard, G. (1991). Frontal cortex contribution to recency judgements. *Neuropsychology, 29*, 601–618.

Mischel, H. N., & Mischel, W. (1983). The development of children's knowledge of self-control strategies. *Child Development, 54*, 603–619.

Mischel, W., Shoda, Y., & Rodriguez, M. L. (1989). Delay of gratification in children. *Science, 244*, 933–938.

Misener, V. L., Luca, P., Azeke, O., Crosbie, J., Waldman, I., Tannock, R., et al. (2004). Linkage of the dopamine receptor D1 gene to attention-deficit/hyperactivity disorder. *Molecular Psychiatry, 9*, 500–509.

Mishkin, M., & Petri, H. L. (1984). Memories and habits: Some implications for the analysis of learning and retention. In N. Butters & L. R. Squire (Eds.), *Neuropsychology of memory* (pp. 287–296). New York: Guilford Press.

Mitchen, S. (1996). *The prehistory of the mind.* London: Thames and London.

Mochi, O., Petrides, M., Doyon, J., Postuma, R. B., Worsley, K., & Dagher, A. (2004). Neural bases of set-shifting deficits in Parkinson's disease. *The Journal of Neuroscience, 24,* 702–710.

Mogenson, G. J., & Huang, Y. H. (1973). The neurobiology of motivated behavior. *Progress in Neurobiology, 1,* 52–83.

Mogenson, G. J., Jones, D. L., & Yim, C. Y. (1980). From motivation to action: Functional interface between the limbic system and the motor system. *Progress in Neurobiology, 14,* 69–97.

Mogenson, G. J., Yang, C. R., & Yim, C. Y. (1991). Influence of dopamine on limbic inputs to the nucleus accumbens. *Annals of the New York Academy of Sciences, 537,* 86–1000.

Montague, P. R., & Berns, G. S. (2002). Neural economics and the biological substrates of valuation. *Neuron, 36,* 265–284.

Montague, P. R., Dayan, P., & Sejnowski, T. J. (1996). A framework for mesenchphalic dopamine systems based on predictive Hebbian learning. *The Journal of Neuroscience, 16,* 1936–1947.

Moore-Ede, M. C. (1986). Physiology of the circadian timing system: Predictive versus reactive homeostasis. *American Journal of Physiology, 250,* 737–752.

Morgan, C. T., & Stellar, E. (1950). Physiological Psychology, New York: McGraw-Hill.

Morgan, M., & LeDoux, J. E. (1995). Differential contribution of dorsal and ventral medial prefrontal cortex to the acquisition and extinction of conditioned fear. *Behavioral Neuroscience, 109,* 681–688.

Morgan, M. A., Schulkin, J., & LeDoux, J. E. (2003). Ventral medial prefrontal cortex and emotional perseveration: the memory for prior extinction training. *Behavioral Brain Research, 156,* 121–130.

Morrison, A. R. (1982). Background to discoveries: Early years in the institute of neurological sciences. *Changing Concepts of the Nervous System.* New York: Academic Press.

Morrow, B. A., Elsworth, J. D., Rasmusson, A. M., & Roth, R. H. (1999). The role of mesoprefrontal dopamine neurons in the acquisition and expression of conditioned fear in the rat. *Neuroscience, 92,* 553–564.

Myers, K. M., & Davis, M. (2002). Behavioral and neural analysis of extinction. *Neuron, 36,* 567–584.

Nakahara, H., Itoh, H., Kawagoe, R., Takikawa, Y., & Hikosaka, O. (2004). Dopamine neurons can represent context dependent error. *Neuron, 41,* 269–280.

Nathan, N. M. L. (1992). *Will and world*. Oxford, UK: Oxford University Press.

Nauta, W. J. H. (1961). The problem of the frontal lobe: A reinterpretation. *Journal of Psychiatric Research, 8*, 167–187.

Nauta, W. J. H., & Domesick, V. B. (1982). Neural associations of the limbic system, In *The neural basis of behavior*. New York: Spectrum.

Nauta, W. J. H., & Freitag, M. (1986). *Fundamental neuroanatomy*. San Francisco: Freeman.

Nauta, W. J. H., Smith, G. P., Faull, R. L. M., & Domesick, V. B. (1978). Efferent connections and nigral afferents of the nucleus accumbens septi in the rat. *Neuroscience, 3*, 385–401.

Nelissen, K., Luppino, G., Vanduffel, W., Rizzolatti, G., & Orban, G. A. (2005). Observing others: Multiple representation in the frontal lobe. *Science, 310*, 333–335.

Neville, R. C. (1974). *The cosmology of freedom*. New Haven, CT: Yale University Press.

Nichols, S., & Stitch, S. P. (2003). *Mindreading*. Oxford: Oxford University.

Nietzsche, F. (1961). Thus spoke Zarathustra (R. J. Hollingdale, Trans.) Baltimore: Penguin Books. (Original work published 1882)

Niv, Y., Duff, M. O., & Dayan, P. (2005). Dopamine uncertainty and TD learning. *Behavioral and Brain Functions, 1*, 1–6.

Norman, D. A., & Shallice, T. (1980). Attention to action: Willed and automatic control of behavior (Report No. 99). University of California at San Diego.

O'Doherty, J., Dayan, P., Schultz, J., Deichmann, R., Friston, K., & Dolan, R. J. (2004). Dissociable roles of ventral and dorsal striatum in instrumental conditioning. *Science, 304*, 452–455.

O'Doherty, J., Kringelbach, M. L., Rolls, E. T., Hornak, J., & Andrews, C. (2001). Abstract reward and punishment representations in the human orbitofrontal cortex. *Nature Neuroscience 4*(1), 95–102.

O'Donnell, P. (1999). Ensemble coding in the nucleus accumbens. *Psychobiology, 27*, 187–197.

Olds, J. (1955). Physiological Mechanisms of Reward. Nebraska Symposium on Motivation.

Olds, J., & Milner, P. (1954). Positive reinforcement produced by electrical stimulation of septal area and other regions of rat brain. *Journal of Comparative and Physiological Psychology, 45*, 419–27.

Oosterlaan, J., Logan, G. D., & Sergeant, J. A. (1998). Response inhibition in AD/HD + CD, anxious, and control children: A meta-analysis of studies with the stop task. *Journal of Child Psychology & Psychiatry & Allied Disciplines. 39*(3), 411–425.

Oswald, L. M., Wong, D. F., McCaul, M., Zhou, Y., Kuwabara, H., Chat, L., et al. (2005). Relationships among ventral striatal dopamine release, cortisol secretion, and subjective responses to amphetamine. *Neuropsychopharmacology, 30,* 821–832

Panksepp, J. (1982). Toward a general psychobiological theory of emotions. *Behavioral and Brain Sciences, 5,* 407–467.

Pardo, J. V., Pardo, P. J., Janer, K. W., & Raichie, M. E. (1990). The anterior cingulated cortex mediates processing selection in the Stroop attentional conflict paradigm. *Proceedings of the National Academy of Sciences, 87,* 256–259.

Parent, A. (1996). Comparative neurobiology of the basal ganglia. New York: Wiley.

Parfit, D. (1984). *Reasons and persons.* Oxford, UK: Oxford University Press.

Parkinson, J. (1817). An Essay on the Shaking Palsy, London: Whittingham and Rowland, for Sherwood, Neely, and Jones. Reprinted 1989 In A. D. Morris, James Parkinson, His Life and Times (pp.152–75). Boston, MA: Birkhauser.

Parrott, W. G., & Schulkin, J. (1993). Neuropsychology and the cognitive nature of emotions. *Cognition and Emotion, 7,* 43–59.

Passingham, R. E (1975). Delayed matching afer selective prefrontal lesions in monkeys. *Brain Research, 92,* 89–102.

Passingham, R. E. (1993). *The frontal lobes and voluntary action.* Oxford Psychology Series, 21. New York: Oxford University Press.

Paus, T. (2001). Primate anterior cingulate cortex: where motor control, drive and cognition interface. *Nature Reviews, Journal of Neuroscience, 2,* 417–424.

Pavlov, I. P. (1927). *Conditioned reflexes. An investigation of the physiological activity of the cerebral cortex.* London: Oxford University Press.

Pears, D. (1985). Motivated Irrationality. Oxford: Oxford University Press.

Peirce, C. S. (1992a). Deduction, induction, and hypothesis, In N. Houser & C. Kloesel (Eds.), *The essential Peirce* (Vol. 1, Chap. 12). Bloomington: Indiana University Press. (original work published in 1878)

Peirce, C. S. (1992b). The doctrine of chances. In N. Houser & C. Kloesel (Eds.), *The essential Peirce* (Vol. 1, Chap. 9). Bloomington: Indiana University Press. (original work published in 1878)

Peirce, C. S. (1992c). The doctrine of necessity examined. In N. Houser & C. Kloesel (Eds.), *The essential Peirce* (Vol. 1, Chap. 22). Bloomington: Indiana University Press. (original work published in 1892)

Peirce, C. S. (1992d). The fixation of belief. In N. Houser & C. Kloesel (Eds.), *The essential Peirce* (Vol. 1, Chap. 7). Bloomington: Indiana University Press. (original work published in 1877)

Pennington, B. F., Van Doornick, W. J., McCabe, L. L., & McCabe, E. R. B. (1985). Neuropsychological deficits in early treated phenylketonuric children. *American Journal Mental Deficiency 89*, 467–474.

Perrett, D., Rolls, E. T., & Caan, W. (1982). Visual neurons responsive to faces in the monkey temporal cortex. *Experimental Brain Research, 47*, 329–342.

Peters, R. S. (1958; 1975). The Concept of Motivation. London: Routledge & Kegan Paul.

Petrides, M. (1998). Specialized systems for the processing of mnemonic information within the primate frontal cortex (pp. 103–130). In A. C. Roberts, T. W. Robbins, & L. Weiskrantz (Eds.), *The prefrontal cortex*. Oxford, UK: Oxford University Press.

Petrides, M., & Pandya, D. N. (1999). Dorsolateral prefrontal cortex: Comparative cytoarchitectonic analysis in the human and the macaque brain and corticocortical connection patterns. *European Journal of Neuroscience, 1*, 1011–1136.

Pezze, M. A., Bast, T., Feldon, J. (2003). Significance of dopamine transmission in the rat medial prefrontal cortex for conditioned fear. *Cerebral Cortex, 312*, 371–380.

Pfaff, D. W. (1999). *Drive, neurobiological and molecular mechanisms of sexual motivation*. Cambridge: MIT Press.

Piaget, J. (1952). *The origins of intelligence in children*. (M. Cook, Trans.). New York: Norton.

Piazza, P. V., & LeMoal, M. (1997). Glucocorticoids as a biological substrate of reward: physiological and pathophysiological implications. *Brain Research Reviews, 25*, 359–372.

Pink, T. (1996). *The psychology of freedom*. Cambridge, UK: Cambridge University Press.

Pinker, S. (1994). *The language instinct*. New York: Morrow.

Pinker, S. (1998). *How the mind works*. New York: Norton.

Pinker, S., & Ullman, T. (2002). The past-tense debate: The past and future of the past tense. *Trends in Cognitive Sciences, 6*(11), 456–464.

Pliszka, S. R., Liotti, M., & Woldorff, M. (2000). Inhibitory control in children with attention-deficit/hyperactivity disorder: Event related potentials identify the processing component and timing of an impaired right-frontal response-inhibition mechanism. *Biological Psychiatry, 48*, 238–246.

Pontieri, F. E., Tanda, G., & Di Chiara, G. (1995). Intravenous cocaine, morphine and amphetamine preferentially increase extracellular dopamine in the shell as compared to the core of the rat's nucleus accumbens. *Proceedings of the National Academy of Sciences USA, 92*, 12304–12308.

Porrino, L. J., & Lyons, D. (2000). Orbital and medial prefrontal cortex and psychostimulant abuse: Studies in animal models. *Cerebral Cortex, 10*, 326–333.

Posada, A., Franck, N., Georgieff, N., & Jeannerod, M. (2001). Anticipating incoming events: An impaired cognitive process in schizophrenia. *Cognition, 81*, 200–225.

Preuss, T. M., Stepniewska, I., & Kaas, J. H. (1996). Movement representation in the dorsal and ventral premotor areas of owl monkeys. A microstimulation study. *Journal of Comparative Neurology, 371*, 649–675.

Pribram, K. H. (1969). The primate prefrontal cortex. *Neuropsychologia, 7*, 259–266.

Price, J. L. (2005). Free will versus survival: Brain systems that underlie intrinsic constraints on behavior. *Journal of Comparative Neurology, 493*, 132–139.

Prinz, W, (2003). Experimental approaches to action. In J. Roessler & N. Eilan (Eds.), *Agency and self-awareness* (pp.) Oxford, UK: Oxford University Press.

Pruessner, J. C., Champagne, F., Meaney, M. J., & Dagher, A. (2004). Dopamine release in response to psychological stress in humans and its relationship to early life maternal care: a PET study. *The Journal of Neuroscience 24*, 2825–2831.

Pujol, J., Torres, L., Deus, J., Cardoner, N., Pifarre, J., Capdevila, A., et al. (1999). Functional magnetic resonance imaging study of frontal lobe activation during word generation in obsessive-compulsive disorder. *Biological Psychiatry, 45*, 891–897.

Pulvermuller, F. (2002). *The neuroscience of language* Oxford, UK: Oxford University Press.

Pulvermuller, F., Shtyrov, Y., & Ilmoniemi, R. (2005). Brain signatures of meaning access in action word recognition. *Journal of Cognitive Neuroscience, 17*, 884–892.

Quirk, G. L., Russo, G. K., Barron, J. L., Lebron, K. (2000). The role of ventromedial prefrontal cortex in the recovery of extinguished fear. *Journal of Neuroscience, 20*, 6225–6231.

Rabinbach, A. (1990). *The Human Motor*. Berkeley: University of California Press.

Rachlin, H. (1995). Self-control: Beyond commitment. *Behavioral and Brain Sciences, 18*, 109–159.

Rachlin H. (2000). *The science of self-control*. Cambridge, MA: Harvard University Press.

Rachlin, H., & Green, L. (1972). Commitment, choice, and self-control. Journal of Experimental Analysis Behavior 17, 15–22.

Rachman, S. (1998). A cognitive theory of obsessions: Elaborations. *Behaviour Research and Therapy, 36*, 385–401.

Rainville, P., Hofbauer, R. K., Paus, T., Duncan, G. H., Bushnell, M. C., & Price, D. D. (1999). Cerebral mechanisms of hypnotic induction and suggestion. *Journal of Cognitive Neuroscience. 11*(1): 110–125.

Rapport, J. L., & Wise, S. P. (1988). Obsessive-compulsive disorder: is it a basal ganglia dysfunction? *Psychopharmacology Bulletin, 24*, 380–384.

Redgrave, P., Prescott, T. J., & Gurney, K. (1999). Is the short-latency dopamine response too short to signal reward error? *Trends in Neural Science, 22*, 146–151.

Rescorla, R. A. (1988). Pavlovian conditioning. *American Psychology, 43*, 151–160.

Rescorla, R. A., & Wagner, A. R. (1972). A theory of Pavlovian conditioning: variations in the effectiveness of reinforcement non-reinforcement. In W. J. Baker & W. Prokasy (Eds.), *Classical conditioning: Current research and theory.* New York: Appleton-Century-Crofts.

Ribot, T. (1894). *The diseases of the will* (4th English ed. from 8th French ed.; M.-M. Snell, Trans.) Chicago: Open Court.

Richter, C. P. (1927). Animal behavior and internal drives. *Quarterly Review of Biology, 2*, 307–343.

Richter, C. P. (1947). Biology of drives. *Journal of Comparative and Physiological Psychology, 40*, 129–134.

Richter, C. P., & Hawkes, C. D. (1939). Increased spontaneous activity and food intake produced in rats by removal of the frontal poles of the brain. *Journal of Neurological Psychiatry, 2*, 231–242.

Rizzolatti, G., Faddiga, L., Fogassi, L., & Gallese, V. (1996). Premotor cortex and the recognition of motor actions. *Cognitive Brain Research, 3*, 131–141.

Rizzolatti, G., Fogassi, L., & Gallese, V. (2000). Cortical mechanisms subserving object grasping and action recognition: A new view on the cortical motor functions. In M. S. Gazzaniga (Ed.), *The new cognitive neurosciences* (2nd ed., pp. 539–552). Cambridge: MIT Press,

Rizzolatti, G., & Luppino, G. (2001). The cortical motor system. *Neuron, 31*, 889–901.

Robbins, T. W. (1996). Dissociating executive functions of the prefrontal cortex. *Philosophical Transactions of the Royal Society, London, Series B., Biological Sciences, 351*, 1463–1470.

Roberts, A. C., & Wallis, J. D. (2000). Inhibitory control and affective processing, the prefrontal cortex. *Cerebral Cortex, 10*, 252–262.

Robertson, G., & Taylor, P. J. (1985). Some cognitive correlates of schizophrenic illnesses. *Psychological Medicine, 15*, 81–98.

Robertson, S., Sandstrom, S. M., Denenberg, V. H., & Palmiter, R. D. (2005). Distinguishing whether dopamine regulates liking, wanting and or action about rewards. *Behavioral Neuroscience, 119,* 5–15.

Robinson, T. E., & Berridge, K. C. (1993). The neural basis of drug craving: An incentive-sensitization theory of addiction. *Brain Research Reviews, 18,* 247–291.

Robinson, T. E., & Kolb, B. (1997). Persistent structural modifications in nucleus accumbens and prefrontal cortex neurons produced by previous experience with amphetamine. *Journal of Neuroscience, 17,* 8491–8497.

Roitman, M. F., Anderson, G., Jones, T. A., & Bernstein, I. L. (2002). Induction of a salt appetite alters dendritic morphology in nucleus accumbens and sensitizes rats to amphetamine. *Journal of Neuroscience, 22.*

Roitman, M. F., Schafe, G. E., Thiele, T. F., & Bernstein, I. L. (1997). Dopamine and sodium appetite: Antagonists suppress sham drinking of NaCl solutions in the rat. *Behavioral Neuroscience, 11,* 606–611.

Roitman, M. F., Wheeler, R. A., & Carelli, R. M. (2005). Nucleus accumbens neurons are innately tuned for rewarding and aversive taste stimuli, encode their predictors, and are linked to motor output. *Neuron, 45,* 587–597.

Rolls, E.T. (1992). Neurophysiological mechanisms underlying face processing within and beyond the temporal cortical visual areas. *Philosophical Transactions of the Royal Society, London, Series B., Biological Sciences, 3355,* 11–21.

Rolls, E.T., & Treves, A. (1998). *Neural Networks and Brain Function.* Oxford: Oxford University Press.

Roozendaal, B., deQuervain, D. F., Ferry, B., Setlow, B., & McGaugh, J. L. (2001). Basolateral amygdala-nucleus acumens interactions in mediating glucocorticoid enhancement of memory consolidation. *Journal of Neuroscience, 21,* 2518–2525.

Rosen, J. B., & Schulkin, J. (2004). Adaptive fear, allostasis and the pathology of anxiety. In J. Schulkin (Ed.), *Allostasis, homeostasis and the costs of physiological adaptation* (pp. 167–227). Cambridge, UK: Cambridge University Press.

Rozin, P. (1998). Evolution and development of brains and cultures. In M. S. Gazzaniga & J. S. Altman (Eds.), *Brain and mind: Evolutionary perspectives.* Strassbourg, France: Human Frontiers Sciences Program.

Rubia, K. et al. (1984). Functional frontalisation with age: mapping neurodevelopmental trajectories with MRI. *Neuroscience and Biobehavioural Reviews, 24*(1), 13–19.

Rubia, K. et al. (1999). Hypofrontality in attention deficit hyperactivity disorder during higher-order motor control: a study with functional MRI. *American Journal of Psychiatry, 156,* 891–896.

Ryle, G. (1949). *The concept of mind.* New York: Harper & Row.

Sabini, J., & Silver, M. (1986). On the captivity of the will: Sympathy, caring, and a moral sense of the human. *Journal for the Theory of Social Behavior, 15*(1), 23–37.

Saper, C. B. (1996). Role of the cerebral cortex and striatum in emotional motor response. In C.B. Saper (Ed.), *Progress in brain research* (pp. 120–158). New York: Elsevier.

Sartre, J.-.P. (1948). *The emotions* (B. Frechtmen, Trans.). New York: Philosophical Library.

Sartre, J.-P. (1956). *Being and nothingness* (H. Barnes, Trans.). New York: Philosophical Library.

Satoh, T., Nakai, S., Sato, T., & Kimura, M. (2003). Correlated coding of motivation and outcome of decision by dopamine neurons. *Journal of Neuroscience, 23,* 9913–9223.

Sawa, A., & Snyder, S. H. (2002). Schizophrenia: Diverse approaches to a complex disease. *Science 296,* 692–685.

Sax, K. W., & Strakowski, S. M. (1998). Enhanced behavioral response to repeated d-amphetamine and personality traits in humans. *Biological Psychiatry, 44*(11), 1192–1195.

Saxena, S., Maidment, K. M., Vapnik, T., Golden, G., Rishwain, M. S. W., Rosen, R. M., et al. (2002). Obsessive-compulsive hoarding: symptom severity and response to multimodal treatment. *Journal of Clinical Psychiatry, 63*(1), 21–27.

Saxena, S., & Rausch, S. L. (2000). Functional neuroimaging and the neuroanatomy of obsessive-compulsive disorder. *Journal Psychiart Clin, North America, 23,* 563–586.

Schachar, R., Mota, V. L., Logan, G. D., Tannock, R., & Klim, P. (2000). Confirmation of an inhibitory control deficit in attention-deficit/hyperactivity disorder. *Journal of Abnormal Child Psychology, 28*(3), 227–235.

Schachar, R., Tannock, R., Marriott, M., & Logan, G. (1995). Deficient inhibitory control in attention deficit hyperactivity disorder. *Journal of Abnormal Child Psychology, 23*(4), 411–437.

Schatzberg, A. F., Rothschild, A. J., Langlais, P. J., Bird, E. D., & Cole, J. O. (1985). A corticosteroid/dopamine hypothesis for psychotic depression and related states. *Journal of Psychiatric Research, 19,* 57–64.

Schelling, T. C. (1992). Self-control. In G. Loewenstein, & J. Elster (Eds.), Choice over time (pp. 167–176). New York: Russell Sage Foundation.

Schmidt, L. A., Fox, N. A., Perez-Edgar, K., Hu, S., & Hamer, D. H. (2001). Association of DRD4 with attention problems in normal childhood development. *Psychiatric Genetics 11,* 25–29.

Schmidt, L. A., Fox, N. A., Rubin, K. J., Sternberg, E. M., Gold, P. W., Smith, C., et al. (1997). Behavioral and neuroendocrine responses in shy children. *Developmental Psychobiology, 30,* 127–140.

Schmidt, L. A., & Schulkin, J. (1999). Extreme Fear, Shyness and Social Phobia. New York: Oxford University Press.

Schopenhauer, A. (1958). *The world as will and representation,* Vols. 1 & 2. (E. F. J. Payne, Trans.). New York: Dover Publications. (Original work published 1818)

Schulkin, J. (1991). *Sodium hunger:* Cambridge: Cambridge University Press.

Schulkin, J. (2000). *Roots of social sensibility and neural function.* Cambridge: MIT Press.

Schulkin, J. (2003). *Rethinking homeostasis.* Cambridge: MIT Press.

Schulkin, J. (2004). *Bodily sensibility: Intelligent action.* Oxford: Oxford University Press.

Schulkin, J., Arnell, P., & Stellar, E. (1985). Running to the taste of salt in mineralocorticoids treated rats. *Hormones and Behavior, 19,* 413–425.

Schultz, W. (1999). The primal basal ganglia and the voluntary control of behaviour. *Journal of Consciousness Studies, 6*(8–9), 31–45.

Schultz, W. (2002). Getting formal with dopamine and reward. *Neuron, 36,* 241–263.

Schultz, W., Dayan, P., & Montague, P. R. (1997). A neural substrate of prediction and reward. *Science, 275,* 1593–1599.

Schwaber, J. S., Kapp, B. S., Higgins, G. A., & Rapp, P. R. (1982). Amygdaloid and basal forebrain direct connections with the nucleus of the solitary tract and the dorsal motor nucleus. *Journal of Neuroscience, 2,* 1424–1438.

Schwartz, C. E., Wright, C. I., Shin, L. M., Kagan, J., & Rauch, S. L. (2003). Inhibited and uninhibited infants "grown up"; adult amygdalar response to novelty. *Science, 300,* 1952–1955.

Schwartz, J. M. (1977). Obsessive-compulsive disorder. *Science & Medicine, 4,* 14–23.

Schwarzkopf, S. B., Mitra, T., & Bruno, J. P. (1992). Sensory gates in rats depleted of dopamine as neonates. *Biological Psychiatry, 31,* 759–773.

Searle, J. R. (1983). Intentionality: An Essay in the Philosophy of Mind. Cambridge: Cambridge University Press.

Searle, J. R. (2001). Rationality in Action. Cambridge: A Bradford Book, MIT Press.

Seidman, L. J., Oscar-Berman, M., Kalinowski, A. G., Ajilore, O., Kremen, W. S., Faraone, S. V., et al. (1995). Experimental and clinical neuropsychological measures of pre-frontal dysfunction in schizophrenia. *Neuropsychology, 9,* 481–490.

Seneca (1969). *Letters from a Stoic.* Translated by R. Campbell. New York: Penguin Books.

Shenton, M. E., Kikinis, R., Jolesz, F. A., Pollak S. D., LeMay, M., Wible, C. G., et al. (1992). Abnormalities of the left temporal lobe and thought disorder in schizophrenia: A quantitative magnetic resonance imaging study. *New England Journal of Medicine*, *327*, 604–612.

Sherrington, C. S. (1893). Further experimental note on the correlation of action of antagonistic muscles. *Proceedings of the Royal Society of London*, *B53*, 407–420.

Sherrington, C. S. (1906/1947). *The Integrative Action of the Nervous System*. New Haven: Yale University Press.

Shidara, M., & Richmond, B. J. (2002). Anterior cingulate: Single neuronal signals related to degree of reward expectancy. *Science*, *296*, 1709–1711.

Shizgal, P. (1999). On the Neural Computation of Utility: Implications from Studies of Brain Stimulation Reward. Chapt. 26. In D. Kahneman, E. Diener, & N. Schwarz (Eds.), *Well-Being: The Foundations of Hedonic Psychology*. New York: Russell Sage Foundation.

Shizgal, P., & Arvanitogiannis, A. (2003). Gambling on dopamine. *Science*, *299*, 301.

Shook, J. R. (2000). The Chicago School of Pragmatism, Vol. 1. History of American Thought

Sidgwick, H. (1907/1981). The Methods of Ethics. Indianapolis: Hackett Publishing Co.

Siegel, E., & Rachlin, H. (1996). Soft commitment: Self-control achieved by response persistence. *Journal of the Experimental Analysis of Behavior*, *64*, 117–128.

Siegel, S., Hinson, R. E., Krank, M. D., & McCully, J. (1982). Heroin "overdose" death: Contribution of drug-associated environmental cues. *Science*, *216*, 436–437.

Sigvardsson, S., Bohman, M., & Cloninger, C. R. (1996). Replication of the Stockholm Adoption Study of alcoholism. Confirmatory cross-fostering analysis. *Archives of General Psychiatry*, *53*(8), 681–687.

Simon, H., Scatton, B., & LeMoal, M. (1980). Dopaminergic A10 neurons are involved in cognitive functions. *Nature*, *286*, 150–151.

Simon, H. A. (1967). Motivational and emotional controls of cognition. *Psychological Review*, *74*, 29–39.

Simon, H. A. (1979). Information processing models of cognition. *Annual Review of Psychology*, *30*, 363–396.

Simon, H. A. (1982). Models of bounded rationality (Vol. 1). Cambridge: MIT Press.

Smilansky, S. (2000). *Free will and illusion*. Oxford, UK: Clarendon Press.

Smith, K. S., Tindell, A. J., Berridge, K. C., & Aldridge, J. W. (2004). Ventral pallidal neuronscode the hedonic enhancement of an NaCl taste after sodium depletion. *Society for Neuroscience,* *437,*

Smith, M. L., Klim, P., & Mallozzi, E. & Hanley, W. B. (1996). A test of the frontal-specificity hypothesis in the cognitive performance of adults with phenylketonuria. *Developmental Neuropsychology,* *12,* 327–341.

Smith, R. (1992). *Inhibition.* Berkeley: University of California Press.

Spanagel, R., & Weiss, F. (1999). The dopamine hypothesis of reward: Past and current status. *Trends in Neurosciences, 22,* 521–527.

Spence, S. A., Brooks, D., Hirsch, S., Liddle, P., Meehan, J., & Grasby, P. (1997). A PET study of Voluntary Movement in Schizophrenic Patients Experiencing Passivity Phenomenon. *Brain,* *120,* 1997–2011.

Spence S. A., & Frith, C. D. (1999). Towards a functional anatomy of volition. *Journal of Consciousness Studies, 6,* 11–29.

Spencer, H. (1855). Principles of Psychology. London: Williams and Norgate.

Spinoza, B. (1955). *On the improvement of the understanding.* New York: Dover Press. (Original work published 1668)

Spitzer, M. (1997). A cognitive neuroscience view of schizophrenic thought disorder. *Schizophrenia Bulletin, 23,* 29–50.

Squire, L., Knowlton, B., & Musen, G. (1993). The structure and organization of memory. *Annual Review of Psychology, 44,* 453–495.

Stein, M. A., Waldman, I. D., Sarampote, C. S., Seymour, K. E., Robb, A. S., Conlon, C., et al. (2005). Dopamine transporter genotype and methylphenidate dose response in children with ADHD. *Neuropsychopharmacology, 30,* 1374–1382.

Stellar, E. (1954). The physiology of motivation. *Psychological Review, 61,* 3–22.

Stellar, E. (1960). Drive and motivation. In J. Field & V. E. Hall (Series Eds.) & H. W. Magoun (Section Ed.), *Handbook of physiology, Section 1, Neurophysiology, Vol. 3.* Washington, DC: American Physiological Society.

Stellar, E., & Corbit, J. D. (1973). Neural control of motivated behavior. *Neurosciences Research Program Bulletin, 11,* 301–410.

Stellar, J. R., & Stellar, E. (1985). *The neurobiology of motivation and reward.* New York: Springer-Verlag.

Sterling, P. (2004). Principles of allostasis: Optimal design, predictive regulation, psychopathology and rational therapeutics. In J. Schulkin (Ed.), *Allostasis, homeostasis and the costs of physio-*

logical adaptation. Cambridge, UK: Cambridge University Press.

Sterling, P., & Eyer, J. (1988). Allostasis: a new paradigm to explain arousal pathology. In S. Fisher, J. Fisher, & J. Reason (Eds.), *Handbook of Life Stress, Cognition and Health.* New York: Wiley.

Stevenson, M. K. (1986). A discounting model for decisions with delayed positive or negative outcomes. *Journal of Experimental Psychology: General, 115,* 131–154.

Stricker, E. M., & Zigmond, M. J. (1974). Effects on homeostasis of intraventricular injections of 6-hydroxydopamine in rats. *Journal of Comparative and Physiological Psychology, 86,* 973–994.

Stroud, S., & Tappolet, C. (2003). *Weakness of will and practical irrationality.* Oxford, UK: Oxford University Press.

Suchan, B., Melde, C., Homberg, V., & Seitz, R. J. (2005). Cingulate cortex activation and competing responses: The role of preparedness for competition. *Behavioral Brain Research, 163,* 219–226.

Sumbre, G., Gutfreund, Y., Fiorito, G., Flash, T., & Hochner, B. (2001). Control of octopus arm extension by a peripheral motor program. *Science, 293,* 1845–1848.

Suri, R. E. (2001). Anticipatory responses of dopamine neurons and cortical neurons reproduced by internal model. *Experimental Brain Research, 140,* 234–240.

Swanson, L. W. (1988). The neural basis of motivated behavior. *Acta Morphol. Neerl.-Scand. 26,* 165–176.

Swanson, L. W. (2000a). Cerebral hemisphere regulation of motivated behavior. *Brain Research, 886,* 113–164.

Swanson, L. W. (2000b). What is the brain? *Trends in Neuroscience, 23*(11), 519–527.

Swanson, L. W. (2003). *Brain architecture.* Oxford, UK: Oxford University Press.

Swanson, L. W. (2005). Anatomy of the soul as reflected in the cerebral hemispheres: neural circuits underlying voluntary control of basic motivated behaviors. *Journal of Comparative Neurology, 493,* 122–131.

Swanson, L. W., & Mogenson, G. J. (1981). Neural mechanisms for the functional coupling of autonomic, endocrine and somatomotor responses in adaptive behavior. *Brain Research Reviews, 3,* 1–34.

Swerdlow, N. R. (2001). Obsessive-compulsive disorder and tic syndromes. *Medical Clinics of North America, 85,* 735–755.

Swerdlow, N. R., & Young, A. B. (2001). Neuropathology in Tourette syndrome: An update. *Advances in Neurology, 85,* 151–161.

Teitelbaum, P. (1971). The encephalization of hunger. *Progress in Physiological Psychology, 4,* 319–350.

Teitelbaum, P. (1977). Levels of integration of the operant. In W. K. Honig & J. E. R. Staddon (Eds.), Handbook of operant behavior. Englewood Cliffs, NJ: Prentice Hall.

Teitelbaum, P., Cheng, M. F., & Rozin, P. (1969). Development of feeding parallels its recovery after hypothalamic damage. *Journal of Comparative and Physiological Psychology, 67*, 430–441.

Tessitore, A., Hariri, A. R., Fera, F., Smith, W. G., Chase, T. N., Hyde, T. M., et al. (2002). Dopamine modulates the response of the human amygdala: a study in Parkinson's disease. *Journal of Neuroscience, 22*, 9099–9103.

Thaler, R. H., & Shefrin, H. (1981). An economic theory of self-control. *Journal of Political Economy 89*, 392–406.

Thorndike, E. J. (1935). The Psychology of Wants, Interests, and Attitudes. New York: Appleton-Century.

Thorpe, W. H. (1963). Leaning and Instinct in Animals. London: Methuen.

Thut, G., Schultz, W., Roelcke, U., Nienhusmeier, M., Missimer, R., Maguire, R. P., et al. (1997). Activation of the human brain by monetary reward. *NeuroReport 8*, 1225–1228.

Tinbergen, N. (1951). *The study of instinct.* Oxford, UK: Clarendon Press.

Toates, F. (1986). *Motivational systems.* New York: Cambridge University Press.

Tobler, P. N., Dickinson, A., & Schultz, W. (2004). Coding of predicted reward omission by dopamine neuronsin a conditioned inhibition paradigm. *Journal of Neuroscience, 22*, 10402–10410.

Tobler, P. N., Florillo, C. D., & Schultz, W. (2005). Adaptive coding of reward value by dopamine neurons. *Science, 307*, 1642–1646.

Todes, D. P. (2002). Pavlov's Physiology Factor. Baltimore: Johns Hopkins University Press.

Tolman, E. C. (1932). Purposive behaviour in animals and men. New York: Century Co.

Tremblay, L., Hollerman, J. R., & Schultz, W. (1998). Modifications of reward expectation-related neuronal activity during learning in primate striatum. *Journal of Neurophysiology, 80*, 964–977.

Tversky, A., & Kahneman, D. (1974). Judgment under uncertainty. *Science 185*, 1124–1130.

Twitchell, T. E. (1954). Sensory factors in purposive movements. *Journal of Neurophysiology, 17*, 239–252.

Tzchentke, T. M. (2000). The medial prefrontal cortex as a part of the brain reward system. *Amino Acids, 19*(1), 211–219.

Tzchentke, T. M. (2001). Pharmacology and behavioral pharmacology of the mesocortical dopamine system. *Progress in Neurobiology, 63*, 241–320.

Ullman, M. T. (2001). A neurocognitive perspective on language: The declarative/procedural model. *Nature Neuroscience, 9,* 266–286.

Ullman, M. T. (2004). Is Broca's area part of a basal ganglia thalamocortical circuit? *Cognition, 92,* 231–270.

Ullman, M. T. et al. (1997). A neural dissociation within language: Evidence that the mental dictionary is part of declarative memory, and that grammatical rules are processed by the procedural system. *Journal of Cognitive Neuroscience, 9,* 266–286.

Ullman, M. T., & Pierpont, E. I. (2005). Specific language impairment is not specific to language: The procedural deficit hypothesis. *Cortex, 41,* 399–433

Ungerleider, L. G., & Mishkin, M. (1982). Two cortical visual systems. In D. Ingle, M. Goodale, & R. Mansfield (Eds.), *Analysis of Visual Behavior.* Cambridge: MIT Press.

Ungerstedt, U. (1971). Adipsia and aphagia after 6-hyrodoxydopamine induced degeneration of the nigro-striatial dopamine system. *Acta Neurologica Scandinavica, 367,* 95–122.

Ungless, M. A., Magill, P. J., & Botam, J. P. (2004). Uniform inhibition of dopamine neurons in the ventral tegmental area by aversive stimuli. *Science, 303,* 2040–2042.

Van den Bree, M. B., Johnson, E. O., Neale, M. C., & Pickens, R. W. (1998). Genetic and environmental influences on drug use and abuse/dependence in male and female twins. *Drug and Alcohol Dependence, 52*(3), 231–241.

Van der Kooy, D., Koda, L. Y., McGinty, J. F., Gerfen, C. R., & Bloom, F. E. (1984). The organization of projections from the cortex, amygdala, and hypothalamus to the nucleus of the solitary tract in rat. *Journal of Comparative Neurology, 224,* 1–24.

Vanderschuren, L. J. M. J., Di Ciano, P., & Everitt, B. J. (2005). Involvement of the dorsal striatum in cue-controlled cocaine seeking, *The Journal of Neuroscience, 25*(38), 8865–8670.

Volkow, N. D., & Fowler, J. S. (2000). Addiction, a disease of compulsion and drive: Involvement of the orbitofronbtal cortex. *Cerebral Cortex, 10,* 318–325.

Volkow, N. D., Wang, G. J., Fischman, M., Foltin, R. W., Fowler, J. S., Abolmradn, N., Vitkun, S., Logan, J., Gatley, S. J., Pappes, N., Hize, & Shea, C. F. (1997). Relationship between subjective effects of cocaine and dopamine transporter occupancy. *Nature, 386,* 827–830.

von Bonin, G. (1960). Some papers on the cerebral cortex. Springfield, IL: Charles C Thomas.

Wakabayashi, K. T., Fields, H. L., & Nicola, S. M. (2004). Dissociation of the role of nucleus accumbens dopamine in responding to reward-predictive cues and waiting for reward. *Behavioral Brain Research, 154,* 19–30.

Waldo, M. C., Adler, L. E., Franks, R., Baker, N., Siegel, C., & Freedman, R. (1986). Sensory gating and schizophrenia. *Biological Psychology, 23,* 108.

Walter, H. (2001). *Neurophilosophy of free will. From libertarian illusions to a concept of natural autonomy* (C. Klohr, Trans.). Cambridge: MIT Press.

Wang, C., Ulbert, S., Schomer, D. L., Marinkovic, K., & Halgren, E. (2005). Responses of human anterior cingulate cortex microdomains to error detection, conflict monitoring, stimulus-response mapping, familiarity and orienting. *Journal of Neuroscience. 25,* 604–613.

Wang, M., Vijayraghavan, S., & Goldman-Rakic, P. S. (2004). Selective D2 receptor actions on the functional circuitry of working memory. *Science, 303,* 853–856

Wegner, D. M. (2002). *The illusion of conscious will.* Cambridge: MIT Press.

Weinberger, D. R. (1988). Schizophrenia and the frontal lobe. *Trends in Neuroscience, 11,* 367–370.

Weiskrantz, L. (1956). Behavioral changes associated with ablation of the amygdaloid complex in monkeys. *Journal of Comparative and Physiological Psychology, 49,* 381–389.

Weissman, D. (2002). *Lost souls.* New York: SUNY.

Wernicke, C. (1874). *Der aphasische Symptomencomplex. Eine psychologische Studie auf anatomischer Basis.* Breslau: Kohn & Weigert.

Wertenbroch, K. (1998). Consumption self-control by rationing purchase quantities of virtue and vice. *Marketing Science, 17,* 317–337.

Whitehead, A. N. (1933, 1967). *Adventure of Ideas.* New York: Free Press.

Williams, B. R., Ponesse, J. S., Schachar, R. J., Logan, G. D., & Tannock, R. (1999). Development of inhibitory control across the life span. *Developmental Psychology, 35*(1), 205–213.

Williams, G. V., & Goldman-Rakic, P. S. (1995). Modulation of memory fields by dopamine D1 receptors in prefrontal cortex. *Nature, 376,* 572–575.

Wingfield, J. (2004). Allostatic load and Life cycles: In J. Schulkin (Ed.), *Allostasis, homeostasis, and the costs of adaptation.* Cambridge, MA: Cambridge University Press.

Wise, R. A. (1987). Sensorimotor modulation and the variable action pattern (VAP): Toward a noncircular definition of drive and motivation. *Psychobiology, 15*(1), 7–20.

Wise, R. A. (2002). Brain reward circuitry: insights from unsensed incentives. *Neuron, 38,* 229–240.

Wise, R. A. (2005). Forebrain substrates of reward and motivation. *Journal of Comparative Neurology, 493,* 115–121.

Wise, R. A., & Bozarth, M. (1987). A psychomotor stimulant theory of addiction. *Psychological Review, 94,* 469–492.

Wise, S. P. (1997). Evolution of neuronal activity during conditional motor learning. In J. R. Bloedel, T. J. Egner, & S. P. Wise (Eds.), *The acquisition of motor behavior in vertebrates.* Cambridge: MIT Press.

Wolf, G. (1969). Innate mechanisms for regulation of sodium appetite. In C. Pfaffmann (Ed.), *Olfaction and taste* (pp. 548–553). New York: Rockefeller University Press.

Worsley, J. N., Moszcynska, A., Falaradeau, P., Kalasinsky, S. K., Schmunk, G., Guttman, M., Furukawa, Y., Ang, L., Adams, V., Reiber, G., Anthony, R. A., Wickman, D., & Kish, S. J. (2000). Dopamine D1 receptor protein is elevated in nucleus accumbens of human, chronic metamphetamine uses. *Molecular Psychiatry, 5,* 664–672.

Young, A. M., Joseph, M. H., & Gray, J. A. (1993). Latent inhibition of conditioned release in rat nucleus accumbens. *Neuroscience, 54,* 5–9.

Zald, D. H., Boileau, I., El-Dearedy, W., Gunn, R., McGlone, F., Dichter, et al. (2004). Dopamine transmission in the human striatum during monetary reward tasks. *Journal of Neuroscience, 24,* 4105–4112.

Author Index

A

Adam, J. E. R., 7
Adey, W. R., 26
Ainslie, G., xvii 9, 90, 93, 94, *95*, 96, 97, 107, 119
Akazawa, T., xv
Aldridge, J. W., 33, 44
Alexander, G. E., 29
Alheid, G. F., 29
Anderson, G., 19
Andreasen, N. C., 83
Anscombe, G. E. M., 112
Aosaki, T., 4
Aragona, B. J., 111
Arbib, M. A., 26
Ariely, D., 100
Aristotle, 65, 115
Arnell, P., 16
Augustine of Hippo, 114
Aurelius, 114
Austin, J. L., 112

B

Badgaiyan, R. D., 97

Badre, D., xvi
Baimoukhametova, D. V., 63
Bain, A., xiii
Bains, J. S., 63
Baker, C., 83
Barch, D. M., 83
Bargh, J. A., 97
Barlow, J. H., 66
Baron, J., 91, 92
Baron-Cohen, S., 41
Barr, L. C., 85
Bast, T., 51
Baumeister, R. Y., 109
Baxter, L. R., 85
Bechara, A., 64, 67, 78, 106
Becker et al., 8
Becker, G. S., 100
Bentham, J., 91
Bergson, H., 12, 17
Berns, G. S., 105
Bernstein, I. L., 19
Berridge, K. C., 7, 14, 16, 17, 18, 25, 33, 66, 67, 71, 75, 77, 78, 85, 102, 105, 110
Berrios, G. E., 80
Berthoz, A., 42, 87

Subject Index

A

Aetycholine, 46
Action and representation of action
    motivation underlaid by, 13
    motor and premotor cortex acti-
        vated by, 5, 40, 87, 118
    parts of brain involved in, 87,
        88
    sensory-motor control and
        prefrontal cortex,
        38–42, 41, 87, 88, 118
Addiction
    central motive states and, 68–70
    choice, reasoning, and self-regu-
        lation, 96–97, 99,
        100–101
    dopamine and, 70–72
        central motive states, 68
        reward, 75–78
        sites of drug action, 72–74
    genetic factors, 78–79
    hormones associated with, 68, 70
    neural mechanisms underlying
        compulsive choices,
        87–89
    reward and, 72, 73, 74–78
    sites of drug action in the brain,
        72–74

    temperamental factors, 79–80
    temptation as element of, 67
    vulnerability to, 75, 78–80
ADHD (attention deficit/hyperactiv-
    ity disorder) and behav-
    ioral inhibition, 61–63, 62
Affiliative bonding, 80, 81
Afflictions. See disease processes
    and trauma
Agency, importance of sense of, 84
Aggressive behavior, novelty-seek-
    ing, and pathology, 79
Alcoholism. See addiction
Amphetamines, 72, 75, 76, 80. See
    also addiction
Amygdala
    addiction, 68, 71–72, 74, 78
    approach systems, 68
    behavioral inhibition and
        self-control, 47, 48, 49,
        54
    central motive states, 18
    choice, reasoning, and self-regu-
        lation, 102–106
    devolution/dissolution of behav-
        ioral regulation in dis-
        ease processes, 42
    dopamine, 8, 71–72